Patch Testing Tips

Jean-Marie Lachapelle • Magnus Bruze
Peter U. Elsner

Editors

Patch Testing Tips

Recommendations from the ICDRG

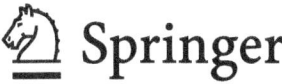 Springer

Editors
Jean-Marie Lachapelle, MD, PhD
Department of Dermatology
Catholic University of Louvain
Cliniques Universitaires Saint-Luc
Brussels
Belgium

Peter U. Elsner, MD, PhD
Department of Dermatology
University Hospital Jena
Jena
Germany

Magnus Bruze, MD, PhD
Department of Occupational
and Environmental Dermatology
Lund University
Malmö
Sweden

ISBN 978-3-642-45394-6   ISBN 978-3-642-45395-3   (eBook)
DOI 10.1007/978-3-642-45395-3
Springer Heidelberg New York Dordrecht London

Library of Congress Control Number: 2014935865

Printed on acid-free paper

Springer is part of Springer Science+Business Media (www.springer.com)

Preface

The idea of writing this book was initiated at the administrative meeting of the ICDRG, held in Malmö during the 11th Congress of the European Society of Contact Dermatitis (ESCD), organized in June 2012 by Magnus Bruze, the new Chairman of the ICDRG. A roundtable and brainstorming among the members led—unanimously—to the choice of the title *Practical Tips*.

Indeed this book is complementary to the previous monograph, *Patch Testing and Prick Testing. A Practical Guide. Official Publication of the ICDRG* (Lachapelle J-M, Maibach HI, editors. Berlin: Springer Verlag; 2012: 218 pages), but it is very different. It is devoted to the latest advances in the field of contact dermato-allergology, based upon our new knowledge of fundamental insights in immunology. The table of contents reflects this tendency.

The main message is that contact dermatitis currently has—in addition to the patch test—a panoply of additional tools of investigation to reach a relevant diagnosis, and this is great.

We are deeply indebted to Howard Maibach, who was and is our master, our mentor, and guide for so many years.

Many tips have been developed in Europe, and we have benefited from the expertise of the ESCD (European Society of Contact Dermatitis) and the EECDRG (Environmental Contact Dermatitis Research Group), which have contributed so much to those advances.

We aim to disseminate them worldwide.

The Editors

Brussels, Belgium   Jean-Marie Lachapelle
Malmö, Sweden   Magnus Bruze
Jena, Germany   Peter U. Elsner

Contents

Contributors

Iris S. Ale, MD Department of Dermatology and Department of Allergy, School of Medicine, Republic University of Uruguay, Montevideo, Uruguay

Klaus Ejner Andersen, MD, DMSc Department of Dermatology and Allergy Centre, Odense University Hospital, University of Southern Denmark, Odense, Denmark

Magnus Bruze, MD, PhD Department of Occupational and Environmental Dermatology, Lund University, Malmö, Sweden

Thomas L. Diepgen, MD, PhD Department of Social Medicine, University Hospital Heidelberg, Heidelberg, Baden-Württemberg, Germany

Peter U. Elsner, MD, PhD Department of Dermatology, University Hospital Jena, Jena, Germany

Hee Chul Eun, MD, PhD Department of Dermatology, Seoul National University Hospital, Seoul, Republic of Korea

Chee Leok Goh, MD, MBBS, MMed (Int Med), MRCP(UK), FRCPE, FAMS National Skin Centre, Singapore, Singapore

An E. Goossens, RPharm, PhD Department of Dermatology, Katholieke Universiteit Leuven, Leuven, Belgium

Jean-Marie Lachapelle, MD, PhD Department of Dermatology, Catholic University of Louvain, Cliniques Universitaires Saint-Luc, Brussels, Belgium

John McFadden, BM, DM Department of Cutaneous Allergy, St. John's Institute of Dermatology, King's College, St. Thomas' Hospital, London, UK

Howard I. Maibach, MD, PhD Department of Dermatology, University of California-San Francisco, San Francisco, CA, USA

Rosemary L. Nixon, BSc (Hons), MBBS, MPH, FACD, FAFOEM Occupational Dermatology Research and Education Centre, Skin and Cancer Foundation Inc., Carlton, VIC, Australia

Denis Sasseville, MD, FRCPC Division of Dermatology,
Department of Medicine, McGill University Health Centre, Royal Victoria Hospital,
Montréal, QC, Canada

Sibylle Schliemann, MD Department of Dermatology, University Hospital Jena,
Jena, Germany

Jessica A. Schweitzer, BS Department of Dermatology, University of California-
San Francisco, San Francisco, CA, USA

Ryan W. Toholka, MBBS (Hons), BMedSci Occupational Dermatology
Research and Education Centre, Skin and Cancer Foundation Inc., Carlton,
VIC, Australia

Patch Testing: A Historical and Current Perspective

Jean-Marie Lachapelle

1.1 Introduction: Claude Bernard and the Birth of Experimental Medicine

Claude Bernard (1813–1878) is universally acknowledged as the founder of experimental medicine (Fig. 1.1). His Magnum opus, written in 1865, "Introduction à l'étude de la médecine expérimentale," was reedited in 1963 [1]. The approach includes six consecutive steps (Table 1.1): observation, hypothesis, experience, results, interpretation, and conclusion, most often abbreviated (OHERIC). Claude Bernard considered that this concise, but abridged, version was incomplete, and he added two footnotes [1]:

- We cannot give off hypotheses without having raised the problem to be solved, because a hypothesis is an answer possible for a question aroused by an observation.
- The experiment is testing the verifiable consequence of the hypothesis.

1.2 Adaptation of Claude Bernard's Methodology to Patch Testing

In my view, when Josef Jadassohn (1863–1936) (Fig. 1.2) performed the first patch test in 1895 at Breslau (now Wroclaw) University, referred to us as "Funktionelle Hautprüfung" [2], it was the very first application in dermatology of the principles of experimental medicine established by Claude Bernard [1]. The "step-by-step" strategy involved in reaching the proper conclusions is still valid today (see Table 1.1). Therefore, initially the patch test was conversely considered an "experimental" and/ or a "diagnostic" tool. It has to be kept in mind that, at that time, before the advent

J.-M. Lachapelle, MD, PhD
Department of Dermatology, Catholic University of Louvain,
Cliniques Universitaires Saint-Luc, 10, Avenue Hippocrate, Brussels B-1200, Belgium
e-mail: jean-marie.lachapelle@uclouvain.be

J.-M. Lachapelle et al. (eds.), *Patch Testing Tips*,
DOI 10.1007/978-3-642-45395-3_1, © Springer-Verlag Berlin Heidelberg 2014

Fig. 1.1 Claude Bernard

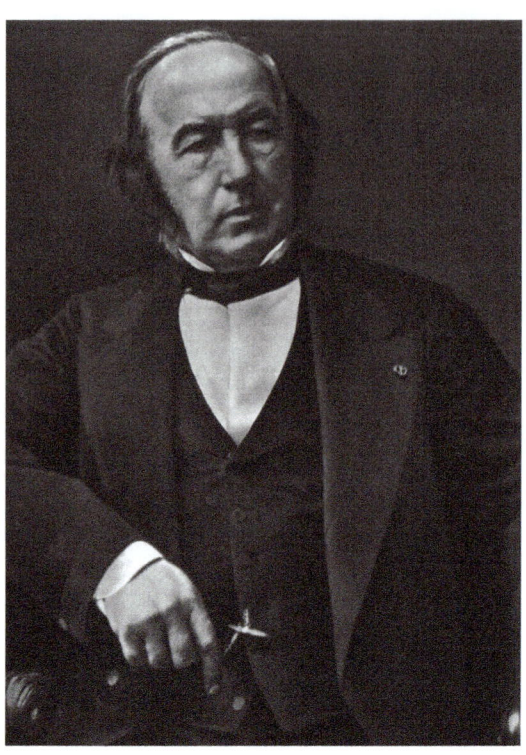

Table 1.1 The steps related to experimental medicine, after Claude Bernard, and their application to patch testing

Steps proposed by Claude Bernard as a trial in the field of experimental medicine	Application of Claude Bernard's methodology to patch testing
Observation	Onset of a skin rash
↓	↓
Hypothesis	Suspected to be either allergic or irritant contact dermatitis, or systemic contact dermatitis, or drug eruption
↓	↓
Experiment	Patch testing as a trial (or a "tool") with the hope to solve the problem
↓	↓
Results	Positive or negative patch tests
↓	↓
Interpretation	Relevance (or non relevance) of positive (or negative) patch tests
↓	↓
Conclusions i.e. « OHERIC »	Conclusions

of the concept of allergy initiated in 1906 by von Pirquet (1874–1924) (Fig. 1.3), the reproducibility of a reaction in a patient by patch testing had no real etiopathogenic meaning. In other words, there was no distinction between irritancy and allergenicity.

Fig. 1.2 Josef Jadassohn

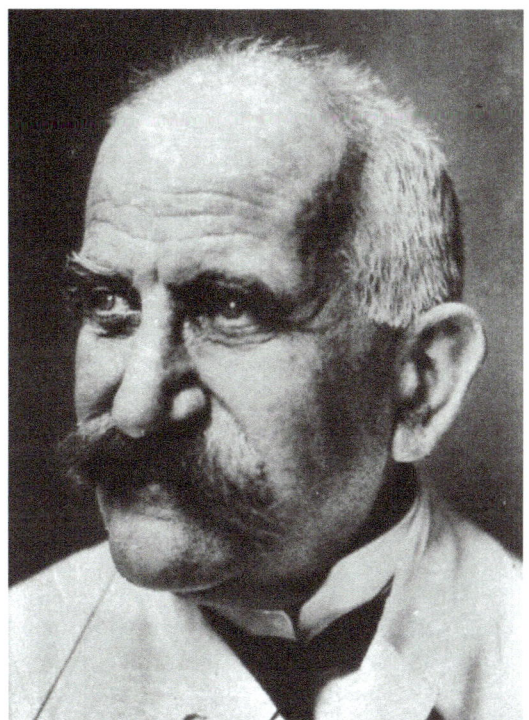

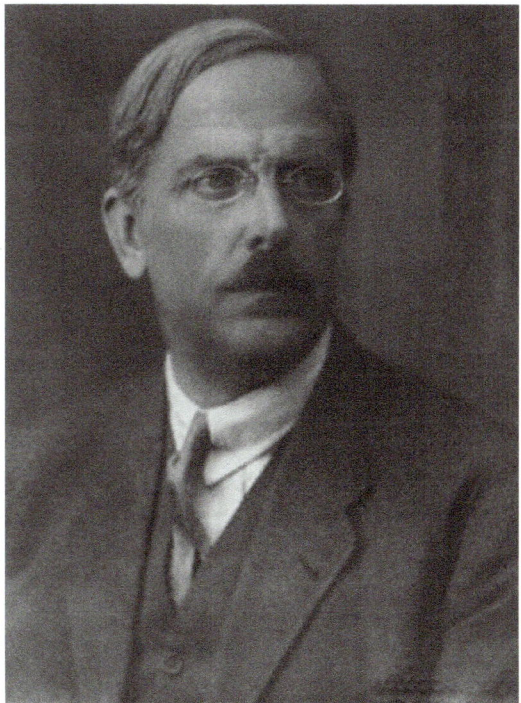

Fig. 1.3 Clemens von Pirquet

1.3 Advances from 1895 to the Creation of the International Contact Dermatitis Research Group (ICDRG)

This period has been extensively reviewed in a recent monograph [3].

A most important contribution came from Clemens von Pirquet (1874–1929), an Austrian scientist and pediatrician who noticed in 1906 that patients who had previously received injections of horse serum or smallpox vaccine had quicker, more severe reactions to a second injection. He coined the word *allergy* to describe this hypersensitivity reaction. Soon after, the observation with smallpox led von Pirquet to realize that tuberculin might lead to a similar type of reaction.

Some papers have been devoted to the scientist and his discoveries [4, 5].

Charles Mantoux (1877–1947) expanded upon von Pirquet's ideas, and the Mantoux test, in which tuberculin is injected into the skin, became a diagnostic test for tuberculosis in 1907. In the field of contact dermato-allergology, the technique of patch testing, initiated by J. Jadassohn, was extensively developed in Zurich by Bruno Bloch (1878–1933); therefore, it is sometimes called the Jadassohn-Bloch technique.

Bloch (Fig. 1.4) was an exceptional teacher and researcher. Indeed, the patch test was one of his lines of clinical research, among many others in different areas of dermatology. He suspected very early the difference between irritant and allergic contact dermatitis. He used the term "idiosyncrasy" [6, 7], which is no longer quoted nowadays; in his view, it was synonymous with allergy. Many dermatologists, coming from different countries, stayed for a rather long period of time in his

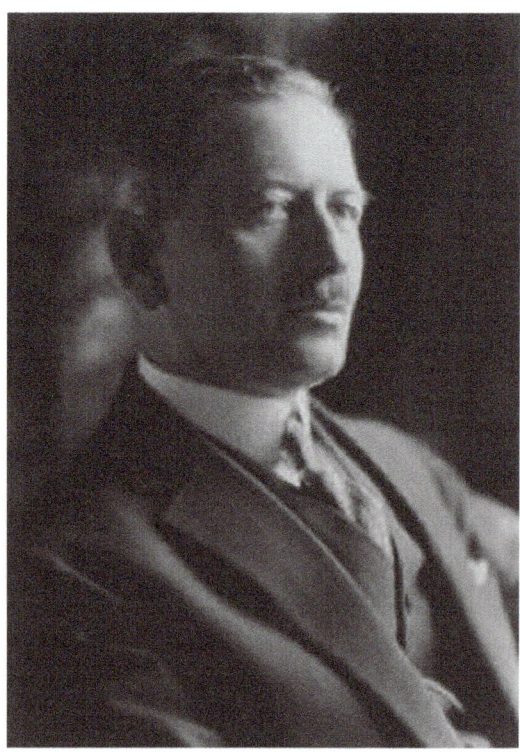

Fig. 1.4 Bruno Bloch

department; among them was Marion Sulzberger (1895–1983) [8], who dissemi-nated and popularized the patch test throughout the United States, and also Poul Bonnevie (1907–1990), who later became Professor of Occupational Medicine in Copenhagen (Fig. 1.5). He introduced the first standard series of patch tests, voca-tionally oriented towards occupational dermatology [9]. Marcussen in 1962 pro-vided a very comprehensive statistical study about the relative frequency of positive and negative patch test results of Bonnevie's standard series [10], unchanged over the years (period of inertia potentially linked with the events of World War II). But the series had become obsolete and did not correspond anymore to the current envi-ronmental conditions.

Apart from Bloch's flourishing school, many publications referring to contact dermatitis and patch testing were recorded in the literature from various countries, most of them of high scientific value [3, 11].

But it is clear that each "patch tester" throughout Europe and the United States had his or her own methodology; all parameters of use (allergens, concentrations, vehicles, reading time etc.) were not codified.

Moreover, it is noteworthy to recall that some individuals proficient in the field were reluctant to use systematically a "standard" or "baseline" series. In particular, Werner Jadassohn (son of Josef) in Geneva [12] and Jean Foussereau in Strasbourg [13] were strenuous opponents of the standard series; ultimately, however, they lost the battle.

It is important, in retrospect, to compare the advantages and disadvantages of a standard series (Table 1.2).

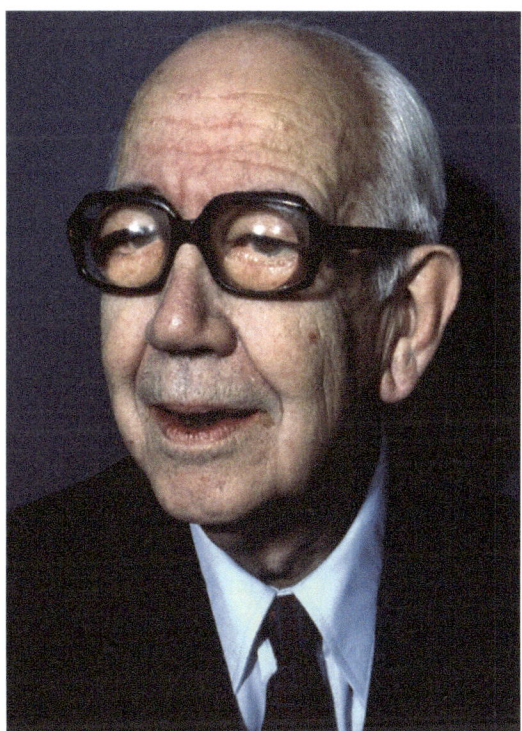

Fig. 1.5 Poul Bonnevie

Table 1.2 Advantages and disadvantages of the systematic use of a standard series

Advantages	Disadvantages [12, 13]
The standard series corresponds to an allergological check-up of each individual patient, as regards the most common allergens encountered in the environment. Positive and negative patch test results map out the allergological profile of the patient;	The standard series can produce a "sleeping" effect on the clinician's attitude. This perverse result is avoided when the standard series is considered as a limited technical tool, representing one of the pieces of a puzzle, to be combined with other means of diagnosis. The general principle to be kept in mind is that the standard series cannot replace a detailed anamnestic (and catamnestic) investigation.
The standard series compensates for anamnestic failures. Even when the clinician tries to record carefully the history of each individual patient, he may omit important events in some cases, despite using a detailed standardized questionnaire. Positive patch test results lead the clinician to ask some additional (retrospective) questions;	Theoretically, application of the standard series could induce an active sensitization to some allergens. Common examples are p-phenylenediamine, primin, or isothiazolinone. The risk, however, is extremely low when testing is performed accordingly to internationally accepted guidelines.
The systematic use of the standard series permits to conduct comparative studies in different countries, thus increasing our knowledge in terms of geographic variations.	

1.4 A Revolutionary Adventure: The Founding of the International Contact Dermatitis Research Group (ICDRG)

The aim was to create a group of dermatologists from different countries, experienced in the field of contact dermato-allergology, who could share the results of their own clinical observations. The ICDRG was informally founded in 1967. Eleven members were elected and met twice a year during three full days, and the presence of everyone was compulsory. The agenda was clearly delineated before each meeting. The members of the "former" ICDRG (as we call it today) were Hans-Jürgen Bandmann (Munich-Schwabing, Germany), Charles D. Calnan (London, Great Britain), Etain Cronin (London, Great Britain), Sigfrid Fregert (Lund, Sweden), Niels Hjörth (Copenhagen, Denmark), Bertil Magnusson (Malmö, Sweden), Howard I. Maibach (San Francisco, United States), Klaus Malten (Nijmegen, the Netherlands), Carlo Meneghini (Bari, Italy), Veikko Pirilä (Helsinki, Finland), and Darrell Wilkinson (High Wycombe, Great Britain).

Niels Hjörth was the leader of the group. He acted as chairman and secretary, but this function was not official, only pragmatic. After each meeting, he wrote the minutes very carefully, without any item escaping his attention.

I was elected full member later on, after Magnusson's sudden death.

The aims of the group were clearly defined [14].

1.5 Major Contributions of the Former ICDRG

1.5.1 Terminology

A precise definition of the terms used in contact dermato-allergology was needed and was achieved by the group [15].

1.5.2 Recommendations About the Patch Testing Methodology: The Early "Tips" in Contact Dermato-Allergology

After long discussions at the biannual meetings, several rules were decided and promulgated. The main recommendations are presented in Table 1.3. For more detailed information, see reference [16].

Table 1.3 Recommendations of the (former) ICDRG related to the patch testing methodology [16]

Choice of a vehicle for the allergens being applied onto the skin	After long discussions, petrolatum was considered the best compromise, because it allows good penetration of the allergens and warrants a long-dated preservation of most allergens kept in the fridge
	The chemical incompatibility between some allergens and petrolatum was pointed out (e.g., formaldehyde, to be dissolved in water)
	The use of organic solvents was abandoned due to their irritant properties
Choice of the site of application	The upper back was considered the best site for the application of the patch tests, in terms of reliability and effectiveness. The decision was based upon earlier experiments conducted by Magnusson et al. [17, 18]
Reading time	A consensus was reached to obtain the most accurate results: two readings (at 48 and 96 h) were ideal, but if only one could be achieved, the advisable reading time was 72 h. A third reading at 7 days was strongly recommended, to reveal positive reactions to either slow-reacting allergens (i.e., neomycin, corticosteroids, etc.) or in the case of "late reactors." It was advocated that one single reading at 48 h had to be banished [16]
Scoring patch test results	The scoring codes of the ICDRG [15] have been universally acknowledged and quoted in many papers
	An update of this scoring index is potentially on the way
Repeating the test when doubtful (±?) results do occur	Questionable patch test results (±? or even + for some allergens) were of concern for the committee
	Repeating patch tests was a judicious step proposed by the group. Allergens were tested at lower concentrations to reach a more precise distinction between irritant and allergic reactions
The standard (baseline) series: the main task of the "former" ICDRG	Due to its undeniable advantages, creating an updated standard series of allergens was a real priority. Collecting the results of their individual clinics, the ICDRG members decided that the choice of the list (20 allergens) was dictated by the 1 % rate (i.e., the general approximate cutoff with 1 % positives in an eczema population in a massive screening)
	It is considered nowadays interesting but outdated
	Additional series were also designed

Table 1.4 Items that were incompletely covered by the (former) ICDRG

1. *Patch test materials*

No instructions were precisely given by the members, as far as the patch test material was concerned. Some used the non-chamber Al-test, whereas others privileged the Finn Chamber. No constraint, but therefore the comparative joint studies were partially biased

2. *The amount of allergen applied to the skin*

In relation to item 1, the amount of allergen applied onto the skin was of no concern, but we have to consider that it was 40 years ago!

3. *The relevance of positive patch tests*

The problem was considered, but members thought that it was difficult to define it precisely, and they did not publish about it. They considered that a complete dermatological "checkup" of the patients was the only way to solve the problem. Anamnestic and catamnestic data, a time-consuming procedure, were in most cases contributory

Table 1.5 Some recommendations of the "new" ICDRG

The repeated open application test (ROAT)	Introduced by Hannuksela and Salo [19], it is an invaluable additional tool of investigation, complementary to the patch test [20, 21]
Revised minimal baseline series	Some papers have been written, referring to the "minimal" baseline series, intended to be used worldwide [22, 23]
Relevance of positive and/or negative patch tests	The problem of the relevance (or non-relevance) of positive and/or negative patch tests is still a difficult issue. Some trails have been traced to help the clinician [24, 25]

1.5.3 Some Items That Were Not Studied Thoroughly by the (Former) ICDRG

Some areas of investigation were incompletely covered at that time. They are listed in Table 1.4.

1.5.4 The Retirement of Members of the "Former" ICDRG and the Revival of the Group

When most of the members retired, some of them advised the dissolution of the group, since they considered that such an adventure was unique and could not be repeated as such. Nevertheless, Howard Maibach decided to take up the challenge, and the revival was a success. At that time, Matti Hannuksela joined the group and developed the repeated open application test (ROAT) [19]. Some of the activities are summarized in Table 1.5.

The list of the current members is presented in ICDRG members.

Table 1.6 The main "tips" from the EECDRG and the ESCD

Appropriate amounts of petrolatum and/or liquids to be applied at patch testing	This is a major contribution for the standardization of patch testing, to be adapted to Finn and/or plastic chambers [26, 27]
Sequential retesting when in doubt of the occurrence of the excited skin syndrome (ESS) in a patient	Development of strategies to solve the problem of EES was considered of primary importance in the patch test readings [28–30]
The allergen bank	An innovative approach, initiated in Odense (Denmark), providing extra-allergens, not distributed in the market, to practicing dermatologists [31, 32]
Reliability of patch testing in drug eruptions	It is a domain that exploded in the last few years. The indications and limitations of patch testing have been progressively pinpointed [33–36]
Ultrasonic bath extracts technology	A very useful tool for extracting allergens from patient-supplied products/materials [37]
Semi-open (or semiocclusive) tests	A very important step in the investigation of difficult cases (patient-supplied products). Halfway between the patch test and the ROAT test [38, 39]
Further advancements in the methodology of the ROAT test	Improvements related to the reliability of the ROAT test: investigations about the site, the size of the test, and the scale of evaluation [20, 21, 40]

1.5.5   The European Environmental and Contact Dermatitis Research Group and the European Society of Contact Dermatitis

In the meantime, contact dermato-allergology, the patch testing procedure, and its additional tools of investigation flourished throughout Europe.

The foundation of the European Environmental and Contact Dermatitis Research Group (EECDRG) and soon after of the European Society of Contact Dermatitis (ESCD) played an important role in these continuous improvements. Moreover, the ESCD decided to create various working subgroups, trying to increase our knowledge about pending problems and to help the clinician in his or her practice. For example, one of the important topics was to evaluate the reliability of patch testing in drug eruptions, among many others. The continual updates in the field were presented in specific sessions during the Congresses organized by the ESCD and published in Contact Dermatitis. By the way, some members of the "new" ICDRG were and/or are members either of the EECDRG or of the ESCD. It is noteworthy that many of the "tips" presented in this monograph have been developed either by the EECDRG or the ESCD (Table 1.6).

The aim of the ICDRG is to disseminate these advances all around the world.

1.5.6 Another Adventure: The TRUE Test

Torkel Fischer and Howard Maibach [41, 42] developed the TRUE Test, a well-known technology of patch testing, as a joint venture with Pharmacia (Uppsala, Sweden) at first and with SmartPractice (Phoenix, Arizona) later on.

A detailed overview of the TRUE Test is presented in our previous book [43].

References

1. Bernard CL. Introduction à l'étude de la médecine expérimentale. Réédition Paris. Paris: Nouvel Office d'Edition; 1963. 371 p.
2. Jadassohn J. Zur Kenntnis der medikamentösen Dermatosen. Verhandlungen der Deutschen Dermatologischen Gesellschaft, Fünfter Congress, Graz, 1895. Wien und Leipzig: Wilhelm Braumüller; 1896. p. 103–90.
3. Lachapelle J-M. Giant steps in patch testing: a historical memoir. Phoenix: Smart-Practice; 2010. 169 p.
4. Huber B. 100 years of allergy: Clemens von Pirquet… his idea of allergy and his immanent concept of disease. Wien Klin Wochenschr. 2006;118:573–9.
5. Huber B. 100 years of allergy: Clemens von Pirquet… his idea of allergy and his immanent concept of disease, 2: The Pirquet concept of allergy. Wien Klin Wochenschr. 2006;118: 718–27.
6. Bloch B. Experimentelle Studien über das Wesen der Jodoformidiosynkrasie. Z Exp Pathol Ther. 1911;9:509–38.
7. Bloch B, Karrer P. Chemische und biologische Untersuchungen über die Primelidiosynkrasie. Beibl Vierteljahrsschr Naturforsch Gesell Zürich. 1927;72:1–25.
8. Sulzberger MB. Three lessons learned in Bloch's clinic. Am J Dermatopathol. 1980;2:321–5.
9. Bonnevie P. Aetiologie und Pathogenese der Ekzemkrankheiten. Klinische Studien über due Ursachen der Ekzeme unter besonderer Berücksichtigung des Diagnostischen Wertes der Ekzemproben. Copenhagen/Barth, Leipzig: Busch; 1939.
10. Marcussen PV. Variations in the incidence of contact hypersensitivities. Trans St Johns Hosp Dermatol Soc. 1962;48:40–9.
11. Sézary A. La pratique des tests épicutanés. Bull Soc Franç Derm Syph. 1935;42:78–83. Bull Soc Franç Derm Syph. 1936;43:641, 1463, 1805. Bull Soc Franç Derm Syph. 1938;45:928, 1872.
12. Jadassohn W. A propos des tests épicutanés "dirigés" dans l'eczéma professionnel. Praxis. 1951;40:50–1.
13. Foussereau J, Benezra C. Les eczémas allergiques professionnels. Paris: Masson; 1970. 507 p.
14. Calnan CD, Fregert S, Magnusson B. The International Contact Dermatitis Research Group. Cutis. 1976;18:708–10.
15. Wilkinson DS, Fregert S, Magnusson B, Bandmann HJ, Calnan CD, Cronin E, et al. Terminology of contact dermatitis. Acta Derm Venereol. 1970;50:287.
16. Lachapelle J-M, Maibach HI. Patch testing and prick testing: a practical guide. Official publication of the ICDRG. 3rd ed. Berlin: Springer; 2012. 218 p.
17. Magnusson B, et al. Standardization of routine patch testing. Report I.Proc Northern Dermatol Soc. Acta Derm Venereol. 1962;42:126–7.
18. Magnusson B, Fregert S, Hjorth N, Hovding G, Pirilä V, Skog E. Routine patch testing. V. Correlations of reactions to the site of dermatitis and the history of the patient. Acta Derm Venereol (Stock). 1969;49:556–63.
19. Hannuksela M, Salo H. The repeated open application test (ROAT). Contact Dermatitis. 1986;14:221–7.

20. Hannuksela M. Sensitivity of various skin sites in the repeated open application test. Am J Contact Dermatitis. 1991;2:102–4.
21. Hannuksela A, Niimäki A, Hannuksela M. Size of the test area does not affect the result of the repeated open application test. Contact Dermatitis. 1993;28:299–300.
22. Lachapelle JM, Ale SI, Freeman S, Frosch PJ, Goh CL, Hannuksela M, et al. Proposal for a revised international standard series of patch tests. Contact Dermatitis. 1997;36:121–3.
23. Alikhan A, Cheng LS, Ale I, Andersen KE, Bruze M, Eun HC, et al. Revised minimal baseline series of the International Contact Dermatitis Research Group: evidence-based approach. Dermatitis. 2011;22:121–2.
24. Ale SI, Maibach HI. Clinical relevance in allergic contact dermatitis. Dermatosen. 1995;43: 119–21.
25. Lachapelle JM. A proposed relevance scoring system for positive allergic patch test reactions: practical implications and limitations. Contact Dermatitis. 1997;36:39–43.
26. Bruze M, Isaksson M, Gruvberger B, Frick-Engfeldt M. Recommendation of appropriate amounts of petrolatum preparation to be applied at patch testing. Contact Dermatitis. 2007;56:281–5.
27. Isaksson M, Gruvberger B, Frick- Engfeldt M, Bruze M. Which test chambers should be used for acetone, ethanol and water solutions when patch testing? Contact Dermatitis. 2007;57:134–6.
28. Maibach HI. The ESS-excited skin syndrome (alias the "angry back"). In: Ring J, Burg G, editors. New trends in allergy. Berlin: Springer; 1981. p. 208–21.
29. Mitchell JC, Maibach HI. The angry back syndrome – the excited skin syndrome. Semin Dermatol. 1982;1:9.
30. Bruynzeel DP, Maibach HI. Excited skin syndrome (angry back). Arch Dermatol. 1986;122: 323–8.
31. Andersen KE. The allergen bank: the idea behind it and the preliminary results with it. Curr Probl Dermatol. 1995;22:1–7.
32. Andersen KE, Rastogi SC, Carlsen L. The allergen bank: a source of extra contact allergens for the dermatologist in practice. Acta Derm Venereol. 1996;76:136–40.
33. Barbaud A, Gonçalo M, Bruynzeel D, Bircher A. Guidelines for performing skin tests with drugs in the investigation of cutaneous adverse drug reactions. Contact Dermatitis. 2001;45:321–8.
34. Barbaud A. Place of drug skin tests. In: Pirchler WJ, editor. Drug hypersensitivity. Basel: Karger; 2007. p. 366–79.
35. Barbaud A. Skin testing in delayed reactions to drugs. Immunol Allergy Clin North Am. 2009;29:517–35.
36. Gonçalo M, Bruynzeel D. Patch testing in adverse drug reactions. In: Johansen JD, Frosch PJ, Lepoittevin J-P, editors. Contact dermatitis. 5th ed. Berlin: Springer; 2011. p. 475–91.
37. Bruze M, Trulsson L, Bendsöe N. Patch testing with ultrasonic bath extracts. Am J Contact Dermat. 1992;3:133–7.
38. Goossens A. Minimizing the risks of missing a contact allergy. Dermatology. 2001;202: 186–9.
39. Goossens A. Alternatives aux patch-tests. Ann Dermatol Venereol. 2009;136:623–5.
40. Johansen JD, Bruze M, Andersen KE, Frosch PJ, Dreier B, White IR, et al. The repeated open application test: suggestions for a scale of evaluation. Contact Dermatitis. 1998;39:95–6.
41. Fischer T, Maibach HI. The thin layer rapid use epicutaneous test (TRUE-Test), a new patch test method with high accuracy. Br J Dermatol. 1985;112:63–8.
42. Fischer T, Maibach HI. Easier patch testing with TRUE Test. J Am Acad Dermatol. 1989;20:447–53.
43. Lachapelle J-M, Maibach HI. True test system. Chapter 6. In: Lachapelle J-M, Maibach HI, editors. Patch testing and prick testing: a practical guide. Official publication of the ICDRG. 3rd ed. Berlin: Springer; 2012. p. 103–11.

Making a Diagnosis

2

Ryan W. Toholka and Rosemary L. Nixon

In this chapter we focus not so much on the interpretation of patch tests, which is a difficult task even for experienced practitioners, but rather how the results of patch testing fit into a diagnostic algorithm. Through patch testing we are able to diagnose a delayed-type hypersensitivity reaction to an allergen(s), or contact allergy. With a history of exposure and of dermatitis occurring in response to skin contact with an allergen, we are able to diagnose allergic contact dermatitis (ACD). An allergen is defined as relevant if it is contributing to the current presentation of dermatitis. Nevertheless, even when a relevant allergen is found on patch testing and the diagnosis of ACD is made, there may yet be other factors contributing to a patient's dermatitis, such as irritant contact dermatitis (ICD) and contact urticaria (CU). Without specifying and subsequently addressing all of the contributing factors of a patient's dermatitis, therapeutic results are likely to be unsatisfactory for the patient and unrewarding for the practitioner.

2.1 Major Differential Diagnoses to Consider in Patients Presenting for Patch Testing

Following in the footsteps of Professor Sigrid Fregert from Sweden and Professor Jean-Marie Lachapelle from Belgium, our approach is to classify factors contributing to dermatitis as being either exogenous or endogenous; however, the balance between these factors will vary in each case [1].

R.W. Toholka, MBBS (Hons), BMedSci
R.L. Nixon, BSc (Hons), MBBS, MPH, FACD, FAFOEM (✉)
Occupational Dermatology Research and Education Centre,
Skin and Cancer Foundation Inc.,
1/80 Drummond Street, Carlton, VIC 3053, Australia
e-mail: ryantoholka@hotmail.com; rnixon@occderm.asn.au

J.-M. Lachapelle et al. (eds.), *Patch Testing Tips*,
DOI 10.1007/978-3-642-45395-3_2, © Springer-Verlag Berlin Heidelberg 2014

2.1.1 Exogenous Conditions

2.1.1.1 Allergic Contact Dermatitis

ACD is mediated by direct contact between an allergen and the skin, resulting in a type IV hypersensitivity response. Patch testing is a practical and informative test used to assist in the diagnosis of this condition, through reproducing skin exposure to allergens.

A sensitizing exposure is required for ACD to occur. After this event, subsequent exposures result in clinical lesions, which tend to develop 24–72 h after the exposure. A crescendo phenomenon is described, whereby lesions slowly increase in severity over days and then slowly resolve. ACD characteristically starts, and is more severe, at sites of contact between the allergen and skin; however, it may extend beyond these areas [1].

Typical examination findings in ACD vary depending upon location and timing. Acute ACD is characterized by erythema and papules, with vesicles and bullae in more severe allergic reactions. In certain areas, such as the eyelids and genitalia, erythema and edema can predominate. Pruritus tends to be the main symptom of ACD [1]. Chronic ACD is typically characterized by lichenification, which may fissure and also be accompanied by vesicles [2].

2.1.1.2 Irritant Contact Dermatitis

ICD is caused by chemicals that directly damage skin structures. ICD results when irritants are in contact with the skin for a sufficient length of time, in sufficiently high concentrations [3]. ICD can occur in any individual, but there is marked inter-individual variation in the threshold for eliciting an irritant reaction [4].

The clinical presentation of ICD is highly variable and influenced by both timing and chronicity.

A "decrescendo phenomenon" is described in acute ICD, whereby the reaction quickly reaches its peak after an exposure and then starts to heal. Lesions tend to appear minutes to hours after exposure. Unlike ACD, acute ICD may appear after the first exposure to a strong irritant [1]. Acute ICD may be painful, burning, or stinging to the patient. It is less commonly pruritic [5].

Examination findings in acute ICD may include erythema, edema, vesicles, bullae, and pustules. With stronger corrosive materials, necrosis and ulceration may also be seen. Lesions are sharply circumscribed to the contact area and generally do not spread elsewhere [1].

Chronic ICD is extremely difficult to distinguish clinically from ACD. Chronic ICD can be painful, burning, stinging, and/or pruritic. Examination typically reveals hyperkeratosis, fissuring, erythema, dryness, and scaling [5].

There is no routine diagnostic test for ICD, and thus, it is considered a diagnosis of exclusion. This is not to imply that it is only diagnosed when other causes are excluded: ICD often coexists with both ACD and endogenous eczema.

2.1.1.3 Contact Urticaria

The contact urticaria syndrome involves a heterogenous group of inflammatory reactions that usually appear within minutes of cutaneous or mucosal contact with the eliciting agent and resolve within a few hours with no residual signs. The reaction may be localized to the skin at the site of contact, have a more generalized effect on the skin, or may have extra-cutaneous effects, such as on the respiratory, gastrointestinal, and vascular systems [6].

Severity can range from very mild "invisible" urticaria, whereby there is only the subjective sensation of itch, to life-threatening anaphylaxis. Prototypical CU presents with a wheal and flare reaction at the site of the contact area [1].

The contact urticaria syndrome is typically divided into three subgroups; non-immunologic CU, immunologic CU, and protein contact dermatitis. Non-immunologic CU is the most common form of CU. Systemic extra-cutaneous reactions are not evoked in this case and no previous sensitization is required [3]. It is caused by substances directly influencing dermal vessel walls or triggering release of vasoactive substances, such as histamine, through non-antibody-mediated means [7]. Immunologic CU is a type 1 hypersensitivity reaction where prior sensitization is required. Secondary contact with the allergen leads to binding of the antigen and IgE on the surface of tissue mast cells and basophils. This triggers the release of multiple inflammatory mediators, including histamine [5]. Testing for immunologic CU may include radioallergosorbent test (RAST) [8] and skin prick testing.

Protein contact dermatitis occurs in the context of recurrent episodes of immunologic CU. It usually presents as hand dermatitis and it also may coexist with other forms of dermatitis. The immediate changes of protein contact dermatitis, such as erythema, wheals, and microvesicles, are often transient and may be difficult to identify on a background of chronic dermatitis. Clinical variants include fingertip dermatitis and chronic paronychia. A detailed history documenting all exposures, especially to proteins in foods and to other immediate allergens such as latex, is essential [1].

2.1.2   Endogenous Conditions

2.1.2.1 Atopic Eczema

Atopic eczema is a pruritic, chronically relapsing skin disease. It is typically characterized by erythematous papules and/or vesicles in a predominantly flexural distribution. The most common symptom is itch, and with chronic scratching and rubbing, lesions become excoriated and lichenified. It is frequently associated with other atopic conditions, asthma, and hay fever, and with a family history of atopic eczema. The condition starts early, with 45 % of all cases starting prior to 6 months of age [9]. When atopic eczema persists into adulthood, chronic lichenified eczema of the hands is a relatively common finding. In these individuals, foot eczema is also common, with almost half having atopic eczema involving their feet [10]. However, the clinical picture may vary widely and the diversity of presentation, combined with the lack of a diagnostic test, may make the diagnosis of atopic eczema difficult to make [11].

2.1.2.2 Nummular/Discoid Eczema

Discoid eczema is characterized by clearly demarcated circular plaques, which are intensely pruritic. It is considered an endogenous form of eczema; however, its etiology is uncertain. Initial lesions tend to be erythematous and exudative but as time progresses, they become scaly and the central erythema clears to become peripheral. Lesions often progress from being discoid to annular and then to dry scaly patches [11].

2.1.2.3 Pompholyx/Dyshidrotic Eczema

This condition is characterized by the sudden onset of clear vesicles without erythema, typically located symmetrically on both palms and/or soles. Lesions may be pruritic and preceded by a hot or prickly sensation. Most episodes resolve within 2–3 weeks but the condition is usually cyclical. The etiology of this condition is also unknown, but an exogenous cause is rarely identified [11]. We prefer to use the term "hand eczema" for this condition rather than define it by its morphology, but semantics in this area are confusing.

2.1.2.4 Hyperkeratotic Palmar Eczema

This is a distinct form of hand eczema and is considered to be endogenous; however, its true etiology remains undefined. It is characterized by hyperkeratotic patches localized to the palms and palmar surface of the fingers, which are prone to fissuring [12].

2.1.2.5 Recurrent Focal Palmar Peeling

This condition is asymptomatic and is characterized by small areas of superficial desquamation of the hands and feet. Lesions first appear as a white macule, expand, and then peel off. There is no fluid within the lesions, and vesicles are not evident [11]. It was previously termed keratolysis exfoliativa.

2.1.2.6 Psoriasis

Psoriasis is a common inflammatory and proliferative condition of the skin. Most commonly it presents as sharply demarcated, erythematous, scaly plaques on extensor surfaces. However, the clinical presentation can be widely varied. Psoriasis occurring on the hands and feet and palmoplantar pustulosis can be particularly difficult to differentiate from contact dermatitis. Nail changes such as pitting, subungual hyperkeratosis, and onycholysis may give the practitioner a clue to the diagnosis of psoriasis. Palmoplantar pustulosis is classified by erythematous and scaly plaques with associated pustules on the palms and/or soles [11].

2.1.3   Other

2.1.3.1 Fungal Infections

Tinea manuum may mimic contact dermatitis. It may cause diffuse scaling on the palms, with prominence in the skin creases. Erythema may or may not be present. It is often unilateral, and associated with tinea pedis, which may give a clue to the diagnosis [1].

2.1.3.2 Photosensitive Dermatoses

A photosensitive dermatosis may mimic airborne contact dermatitis. This is important to consider in patients who present with dermatitis of the face, neck, lower arms, and dorsum of the hands. Causes particularly include drug hypersensitivity.

Porphyria cutanea tarda may involve the dorsum of the hands with characteristic erosions, blisters, skin fragility, and milia [8].

2.2 Diagnostic Pathway

2.2.1 History

2.2.1.1 History of Presenting Complaint

A thorough history is integral to making the diagnosis of all conditions, with particular reference to exposures including chemicals, water and skin contactants such as gloves, and skin cleansers (Table 2.1).

2.2.1.2 Exposure History

When considering the diagnosis of contact dermatitis, it is important to accurately determine all of the substances that come in contact with the patient's skin.

Table 2.1 History of presenting complaint

Features of presenting complaint	Questions
Site	Where did the rash start? This may give a clue as to the nature of the initial allergen. Did the rash spread subsequently? What areas of the body are affected by the rash?
Symptoms	Is it itchy?
Onset	When did the rash start? Are there any new exposures that the patient can associate with development of the rash? How long after the exposure did the rash start?
Time course	How has the rash progressed? Has it spread to other areas?
Morphology	What is the nature of the rash? Does the description sound eczematous?
Aggravating factors	Are there any exposures or factors that make the rash worse? Does work generally or any particular tasks at work exacerbate the condition?
Relieving factors	What has the patient found improves their rash?
Response to treatment	What treatments have been tried and have they helped? Were oral corticosteroids required?
Work relatedness	Does time away from work help? How long does it take to improve?
Associated features	Has the patient experienced any breathing difficulties or lip or tongue swelling?
Severity	A rating system out of 10, scored by both patient and doctor, can help assess relative severity. The rash may have improved prior to assessment. It also aids in monitoring progress at future visits

Table 2.2 Exposure history

Personal exposures	Hand washing – frequency denoting wet work exposure, soaps, liquid soaps, hand cleaners
	Hair products – shampoo, conditioner, dyes, gels, waxes, sprays
	Makeup – facial products, eye products, lip products, nail products
	Fragrances – colognes, perfume, deodorants
	Body washing – frequency, soaps, liquid soaps
	Sunscreens
	Moist wipes
	Shaving cream
	Moisturizers
	Topical medicaments
	Use of reusable or disposable gloves at home
	Jewelry
Occupational exposures	Which substances does the patient come in direct skin contact with? It is important to ascertain specific constituents of chemicals, in particular assessing for likely allergens or irritants, through review of safety data sheets. It is important to note that allergy may develop at any stage of exposure to an allergen. The causative allergen may not necessarily be a new exposure: allergies can start at any stage
	What personal protective equipment (PPE) is used? Is it always used?
	Have there been times when there has been an accidental spill of chemicals or PPE has failed?
	What types of gloves are used? Disposable or reusable? Powdered? How often? For what tasks?
	Which substances may be airborne?
	Does the skin improve when the worker is away from work? Once exposures have been determined, the association between exposures and the skin condition needs to be explored. Does the condition worsen on return to work? How long does it take to get worse? Has anyone else at work had skin problems?

Knowledge of potential allergens is essential to direct appropriate patch testing, and it is also important to document exposures to skin irritants.

Exposures may be classified as personal and occupational (Table 2.2).

2.2.1.3 Past Medical History

- Atopy: Atopy includes atopic eczema and/or asthma and/or hay fever. There are many definitions but essentially the determination of atopy involves establishing a background of atopic eczema and/or asthma and/or hay fever. Atopy is a known risk factor for occupational contact dermatitis [13].
- Dermatological conditions.
- Medical/surgical conditions.

2.2.1.4 Family History

- Atopy: A prospective cohort study of infants from birth to 4 years of age emphasized family history as an important risk factor for atopic eczema, with 38 % of children with one parent with a history of atopy developing atopic eczema and 50 % of those whose parents both had history of atopy [14].

- Psoriasis: Family history conveys a significant risk of developing psoriasis. A Serbian and Montenegro study showed that one is more likely to develop psoriasis if a family history of psoriasis is present, with an odds ratio of 30 in men and 17 in women [15]. This is consistent with an Italian study, which quoted a similar odds ratio of 19 for the development of psoriasis, where there was a family history [16].

2.2.1.5 Medications
- Medications used for the treatment of skin conditions, including both topical and systemic treatments.
- Other medications.
- Have there been any new medications, which may have coincided with the development of the patient's skin condition?
- Nonprescription medications, natural remedies, and herbs.
- Is the patient on any immunomodulatory or oral corticosteroids which may impact upon patch testing?

2.2.1.6 Allergies
- This includes allergies to medications and food and immediate reactions such as animal, pollen, and house dust mite allergy.
- History of contact allergy such as to nickel, fragrance, and sticking plaster. It is suspected that individuals with known ACD are more likely to develop further sensitivities and that the number of contact allergies may be regarded as an indirect expression of the degree of inherent susceptibility to become sensitized [17].

2.2.1.7 Smoking
- Smoking has been shown to convey a significant risk for the development of hand eczema [18].

2.3   Examination

A thorough skin examination can give multiple clues to a patient's diagnosis. It is important to always consider the relationship between the site of dermatitis and particular exposures (Table 2.3).

Although examination can direct the practitioner to the likely cause of a patient's skin condition, too much focus on morphology can narrow the practitioner's mind to other diagnoses. There are a variety of presentations of ACD, ICD, and endogenous forms of eczema, all with significant overlap. There are no absolutes in regard to clinical signs and a diagnosis. Pompholyx or dyshidrotic eczema is characterized by typical vesicles bunched on palmar skin or lateral aspects of the fingers; however, ACD can be a contributing factor, as was evident in an Indian study in which 40 % of patients who presented with pompholyx had a positive reaction to one or more

Table 2.3 Examination of the skin

Site	Considerations
Scalp	Involvement may provide evidence for the diagnosis of ACD from hair products; alternatively, psoriasis and seborrheic dermatitis may involve the scalp
Face	This is a common site for contact dermatitis, with eyelid involvement often found in allergic contact dermatitis [3]. It can be difficult to differentiate between an airborne contact dermatitis and a photosensitive dermatosis because the areas of involvement are similar. It is important to examine the eyelids, underneath the chin, and posterior auricular areas, which may be involved in airborne contact dermatitis but tend to be spared in a photosensitive dermatosis
Trunk	Involvement may point to an endogenous process as there is generally less direct exposure to allergens on the trunk
Hands/ forearms	These are the most common sites for exposures to irritants and allergens
Feet	Involvement may indicate allergic contact dermatitis from footwear, such as to chromate found in leather, or an endogenous form of eczema or psoriasis

allergens on patch testing [19]. Paronychia is most commonly associated with ICD; however, there are reports of ACD and CU presenting with paronychia [20, 21]. It is important to patch test patients with persistent dermatitis, even if the morphology does not suggest an allergic cause.

2.4 Investigations

See Table 2.4.

2.5 Diagnosis

Explaining specific diagnoses to the patient is essential. The use of the holistic term "hand eczema," while helpful for self-reported epidemiological studies [26], conveys minimal information to the patient themselves. A 2009 report attempted to classify patients into six subgroups: ACD, ICD, atopic hand eczema, discoid hand eczema, vesicular hand eczema, and hyperkeratotic hand eczema [27]. However, in practice, there may be multiple contributing factors to the same patient's skin condition, and ACD, ICD, CU, and an underlying endogenous form of eczema may all coexist. Patients need to appreciate the complexity of the diagnostic process and require a specific, tailored list of all of the factors contributing to their skin condition. Their management plan needs to address all of these factors.

Figure 2.1 is an algorithm of the diagnostic journey that we discuss with the patient following patch testing. It is annotated during the final consultation with the diagnoses made, in order of perceived relevance to their specific presentation. Highlighting the contributing factors and also the complexity of this process is pivotal for the patient's understanding of their condition and allows them to be actively involved in their management (e.g., by assisting in searching for sources of exposure to allergens).

Table 2.4 Investigation

Investigation	Considerations
Patch testing	It is important to patch test all individuals with a persistent eczematous skin condition, at least to exclude the possibility of ACD. Patch testing should be done to a location-specific baseline series of the commonly encountered contact allergens; other series relevant to exposure, such as hairdressing allergens; and appropriately diluted samples of the patient's own products
Radioallergosorbent testing (RAST)	Latex – this is important if the patient has any exposure to latex. Patients wearing reusable, not just disposable, gloves may develop latex allergy [22]. Measuring serum-specific latex IgE does not expose the patient to the latex protein and is an appropriate screen, prior to progressing to prick testing, if required
	Other specific IgE – consider if there is a good history of immediate reactions to a certain allergen. In our experience, reactions to house dust mites and to animals have most relevance [23]
Total IgE	Although this is not a diagnostic test, it can be helpful in assessing a patient's atopic predisposition and appears to correlate with the degree of atopic eczema [24]. It can therefore assist with the future direction of treatment. In our experience, atopics with very high IgE are more likely to require more aggressive immunosuppressive therapy for their condition
Repeated open application test (ROAT)	This is not routine, yet can be a useful adjunct to patch testing. Test substances are applied to the same area of skin twice daily for 7 days or until a reaction occurs if prior to 7 days [1]. It can be of particular help in clarifying doubtful and weak, yet suspicious, patch test reactions. It may assist in confirming whether a specific product contains a reagent in a sufficient enough concentration to elicit ACD
Skin prick testing	This is used to diagnose ICU along with RAST tests. This is important to consider if the clinical presentation is consistent with an immediate reaction and is particularly important when allergens are not available for RAST tests. On the other hand, there is a lack of standardization regarding the concentration used for testing many contact urticants
Testing for non-immunologic contact urticaria	This is another area where the literature is scant. In an open test, a small amount of a test substance is applied to the volar aspect of intact skin of the forearm for 30–45 min [3]
Fungal scrapings	Consider with scaly dermatoses of the hands and feet to exclude fungal infection
Skin biopsy	If the morphology of the rash does not clearly indicate an eczematous process, a biopsy can help in the diagnostic process. A biopsy, however, is not reliable in differentiating between an endogenous and exogenous cause of dermatitis [25]

At our occupational contact dermatitis clinic in Melbourne, Australia, from July 2000 to June 2010, 64.5 % of all patients with occupational contact dermatitis had more than one factor identified as contributing to their presentation (unpublished data submitted for publication).

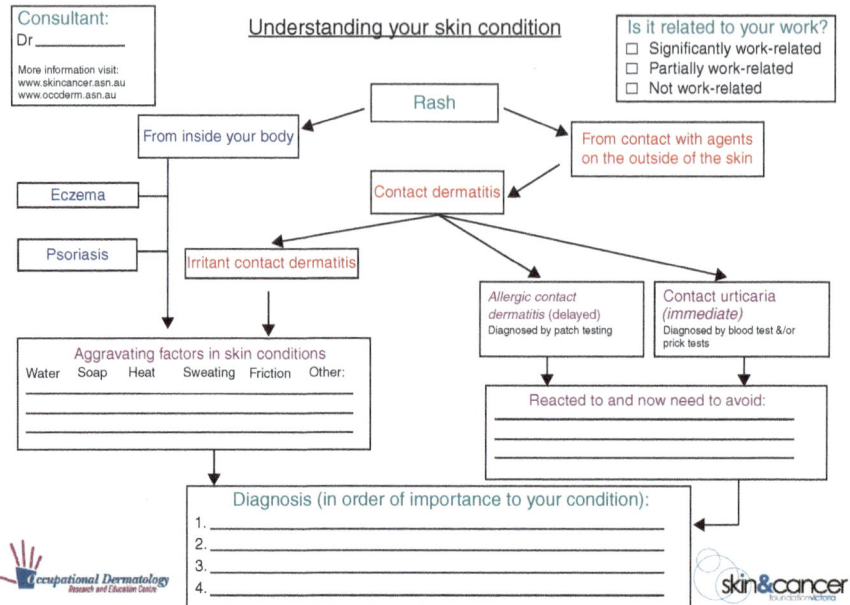

Fig. 2.1 Algorithm of the diagnostic journey

2.5.1 Atopics and Multiple Diagnoses

It is especially important to consider multiple diagnoses in atopic individuals. In the unpublished study mentioned above, the proportion of atopic individuals with multiple diagnoses compared to non-atopic individuals was significantly higher: 76.6 % versus 52.1 % $p=0.0001$. Of course, many of the atopics were also diagnosed with atopic eczema, which contributed to their number of diagnoses. However, they often experienced CU as well as contact dermatitis.

A personal history of atopic eczema is a significant risk factor for the development of occupational dermatitis [13] and of contact urticaria [28]. There is also an association between atopy and protein contact dermatitis, with one study documenting approximately 50 % of cases of protein contact dermatitis having concomitant atopy [29].

Cases have also been reported whereby it is believed occupational contact dermatitis, particularly ICD, has triggered generalized eczema in atopic individuals [30].

2.5.2 Irritant Contact Dermatitis Increases Susceptibility to ACD

ICD often plays a role, even in the context where relevant allergens have been found and the patient diagnosed with ACD as well. ICD causes skin barrier damage and allows increased allergen penetration. It thus often precedes and facilitates ACD [5].

Hairdressers, for example, are often initially exposed to irritants including wet work and then subsequently to potent allergens, including paraphenylenediamine (hair dye), ammonium persulfate (hairdressing bleach), and glyceryl monothioglycolate (perming solution) [31].

2.6   Follow-up

After the patient has completed the patch testing process and diagnoses have been made, appropriate follow-up is essential. Once the patient has been able to implement particular avoidance measures, it becomes easier to assess the contribution that certain factors have played in the causation of their condition. This is commonly encountered when a relevant allergen is found, yet avoidance of this allergen fails to lead to complete improvement in the patient's dermatitis, as the contribution of ICD has been underestimated. The diagnostic journey is a dynamic process and needs regular review.

The patient is also bombarded with a considerable amount of information during patch testing. On review, it is important to revise the initial diagnoses and management plan with the patient while ensuring that treatment is appropriate and being adhered to. In a study of 230 patients contacted 2–9 years after their diagnosis of occupational contact dermatitis, only 33 % could correctly identify their diagnosis. These patients were more likely to report improvement and/or clearance of their symptoms [32]. In a trial of 424 patients, 172 received extra education at the time of their diagnosis from a specifically trained nurse. In patients with a diagnosis of ICD, the prognosis was significantly improved for those who received extra education [33].

There are multiple reasons as to why a patient's dermatitis may have failed to improve with the initial management plan. In a study looking specifically at clinical outcomes of patients diagnosed with occupational contact dermatitis, 64 % of patients had some degree of ongoing dermatitis [34]. The most common causes for lack of improvement were continued exposure despite the patient being aware of this exposure, a new skin condition, a preexisting skin condition, and a new non-occupational exposure. In some cases where there was no obvious cause for the present and ongoing dermatitis, yet there was a clear initial occupational causation, the patients were diagnosed with persistent post-occupational dermatitis (PPOD) [34]. In PPOD, the dermatitis is assessed as initially being work related but fails to resolve with appropriate avoidance of causative allergens and irritants [35].

Conclusion

The assessment of a patient with suspected ACD undergoing patch testing is a complex and dynamic process. More than one factor may be contributing to their dermatitis. If positive allergen(s) is found, providing the patient with detailed information about the allergen(s) and where they may be encountered is essential. Often in our clinic, it is the patient themselves who identify the source, and thus relevance, of a particular allergen. On the other hand, some positive reactions may have no current clinical relevance. Additional investigations may need to be undertaken in order to diagnose CU, and latex is still an important cause of this in our setting. Finally, addressing all the factors contributing in each case is important to maximize patients' outcomes.

Practical Tips
- Make a diagnosis of all the factors contributing to a patient's skin condition.
- Remember that latex allergy can be contributed by use of reusable rubber gloves.
- Involve the patient in the diagnostic process, and involve them in searching for possible exposures to allergens identified on patch testing.
- Following up patients can assist in refining the diagnosis made at the time of patch testing.

References

1. Lachapelle JM, Maibach HI, editors. Patch testing and prick testing. 3rd ed. Berlin: Springer; 2012.
2. Wolff K, Goldsmith LA, Katz SI, Gilchrist B, Paller A, Leffell DJ, editors. Fitzpatrick's dermatology in general medicine. 7th ed. New York: McGraw Hill; 2008.
3. Rietschel RL, Fowler Jr JF, editors. Fisher's contact dermatitis. 6th ed. Philadelphia: Lippincott Williams and Wilkins; 2008.
4. Judge MR, Griffiths HA, Basketter DA, White IR, Rycroft RJ, McFadden JP. Variation in response of human skin to irritant challenge. Contact Dermatitis. 1996;34:115–7.
5. Frosche PJ, Menne T, Lepoittevin JP, editors. Contact dermatitis. 4th ed. Berlin: Springer; 2006.
6. Gimenez-Arnau A, Maurer M, De La Cuadra J, Maibach H. Immediate contact skin reactions, an update of contact urticaria, contact urticaria syndrome and protein contact dermatitis – "a never ending story". Eur J Dermatol. 2010;20:552–62. http://www.ncbi.nlm.nih.gov/pubmed/20732848.
7. Lahti A. Non-immunologic contact urticaria. Acta Derm Venereol Suppl (Stock). 1980;Suppl 91:1–49.
8. Makhija M, O'Gorman MR. Chapter 31: Common in vitro tests for allergy and immunology. Allergy Asthma Proc. 2012;33 Suppl 1:S108–11.
9. Sohn A, Frankel A, Patel RV, Goldenberg G. Eczema. Mt Sinai J Med. 2011;78:730–9.
10. Lee HJ, Ha SJ, Ahn WK, Kim D, Park YM, Byun DG, et al. Clinical evaluation of atopic hand-foot dermatitis. Pediatr Dermatol. 2001;18:102–6.
11. Burns T, Breathnach S, Cox N, Griffiths C. Rook's textbook of dermatology. 8th ed. West Sussex: John Wiley and Sons; 2010.
12. Hersle K, Mobacken H. Hyperkeratotic dermatitis of the palms. Br J Dermatol. 1982;107:195–201.
13. Dickel H, Bruckner TM, Schmidt A, Diepgen TL. Impact of atopic skin diathesis on occupational skin disease incidence in a working population. J Invest Dermatol. 2003;121:37–40.
14. Böhme M, Wickman M, Lennart Nordvall S, Svartengren M, Wahlgren CF. Family history and risk of atopic dermatitis in children up to 4 years. Clin Exp Allergy. 2003;33:1226–31.

15. Jankovic S, Raznatovic M, Marinkovic J, Jankovic J, Maksimovic N. Risk factors for psoriasis: a case–control study. J Dermatol. 2009;36:328–34.
16. Naldi L, Parazzini F, Brevi A, Peserico A, Veller Fornasa C, et al. Family history, smoking habits, alcohol consumption and risk of psoriasis. Br J Dermatol. 1992;127:212–7.
17. Carlsen BC, Andersen KE, Menné T, Johansen JD. Patients with multiple contact allergies: a review. Contact Dermatitis. 2008;58:1–8.
18. Thyssen JP, Linneberg A, Menné T, Nielsen NH, Johansen JD. The effect of tobacco smoking and alcohol consumption on the prevalence of self-reported hand eczema: a cross-sectional population-based study. Br J Dermatol. 2010;162:619–26.
19. Jain VK, Aggarwal K, Passi S, Gupta S. Role of contact allergens in pompholyx. J Dermatol. 2004;31:188–93.
20. Kanerva L, Henriks-Eckerman ML, Estlander T, Jolanki R. Dentists's occupational allergic paronychia and contact dermatitis caused by acrylics. Eur J Dermatol. 1997;7:177–80.
21. Tosti A, Guerra L, Morelli R, Bardazzi F, Fanti PA. Role of food in the pathogenesis of chronic paronychia. J Am Acad Dermatol. 1992;27:706–10.
22. Bhahba F, Palmer A, Nixon R. Are reusable rubber gloves associated with latex allergy? Contact Dermatitis. 2012;67:381–2.
23. Bhaba F, Nixon R. Occupational exposure to laboratory animals causing a severe exacerbation of atopic eczema. Australas J Dermatol. 2012;53:154–5.
24. Laske N, Niggemann B. Does the severity of atopic dermatitis correlate with serum IgE levels? Pediatr Allergy Immunol. 2004;15:86–8.
25. Phelps RG, Miller MK, Singh F. The varieties of "eczema": clinicopathologic correlation. Clin Dermatol. 2003;21:95–100.
26. Meding B, Swanbeck G. Predictive factors for hand eczema. Contact Dermatitis. 1990;23:154–61.
27. Diepgen TL, Andersen KE, Brandao FM, Bruze M, Bruynzeel DP, Frosch P, et al. Hand eczema classification: a cross-sectional, multicentre study of the aetiology and morphology of hand eczema. Br J Dermatol. 2009;160:353–8.
28. Williams JDL, Lee AYL, Matheson MC, Frowen KE, Noonan AM, Nixon RL. Occupational contact urticaria: Australian data. Br J Dermatol. 2008;159:125–31.
29. Doutre MS. Occupational contact urticaria and protein contact dermatitis. Eur J Dermatol. 2005;15:419–24.
30. Williams J, Cahill J, Nixon R. Occupational autoeczematization or atopic eczema precipitated by occupational contact dermatitis? Contact Dermatitis. 2007;56:21–6.
31. Lysdal SH, Søsted H, Andersen KE, Johansen JD. Hand eczema in hairdressers: a Danish register-based study of the prevalence of hand eczema and its career consequences. Contact Dermatitis. 2011;65:151–8.
32. Holness DL, Nethercott JR. Is a worker's understanding of their diagnosis an important determinant of outcome in occupational contact dermatitis? Contact Dermatitis. 1991;25:296–301.
33. Kalimo K, Kautiainen H, Niskanen T, Niemi L. 'Eczema school' to improve compliance in an occupational dermatology clinic. Contact Dermatitis. 1999;41:315–9.
34. Nixon R, Williams J, Matheson M, Palmer A, Frowen K, Dharmage S. Describing outcomes in occupational dermatitis. Recent Adv Recent Updat. 2010;11:71–82.
35. Wall L, Gebauer KA. A follow-up study of occupational skin disease in Western Australia. Contact Dermatitis. 1991;24:241–3.

Pitfalls and Errors in Patch Testing: Suggestions for Quality Assurance

Peter U. Elsner and Sibylle Schliemann

3.1 Introduction

Patch testing is a biological test, and as all biological tests, it depends on many objective variables that may affect its validity. Furthermore, as all medical procedures, it is also subject to possible mistakes and errors. While medical error reporting has improved in recent years, the quality of error reporting that might be used for preventive purposes in the medical profession is still far below the standard found in aviation [1]. No statistical data are available for the kind of errors encountered in patch testing and their incidence. A recent report focussed on medical professional liability claims against dermatologists does not indicate if claims have been brought forward due to errors in patch testing [2]. Even anecdotal reports on pitfalls and errors in patch testing are rare. Standard textbooks on patch testing do not provide recommendations for quality assurance in a structured way. Thus, the present compilation of pitfalls and error sources in patch testing is mainly based on personal experience, either from own clinical practice or from expert opinions in occupational dermatology cases where patch test protocols are frequently reviewed.

3.2 Pitfalls in Patient Selection

Patch testing may reveal the cause of allergic contact dermatitis, but positive results may be irrelevant in patients with other skin diseases or in persons with no skin diseases at all (e.g., patients with psoriasis run the same risk of showing a positive patch test as the general population). One has to be aware that like any medical test,

P.U. Elsner, MD, PhD (✉) • S. Schliemann, MD
Department of Dermatology, University Hospital Jena,
Erfurter Str. 35, Jena 07743, Germany
e-mail: elsner@derma-jena.de; schliemann@derma-jena.de

J.-M. Lachapelle et al. (eds.), *Patch Testing Tips*,
DOI 10.1007/978-3-642-45395-3_3, © Springer-Verlag Berlin Heidelberg 2014

patch testing has limited sensitivity and specificity: Nethercott estimated a sensitivity of 70 % and a specificity of 70 % [3].

When this valuable diagnostic tool is used in asymptomatic persons without medical diagnostic indication, clinical epidemiology teaches us that the risk of false-positive tests is higher than in persons actually suffering from contact dermatitis. A recent study by the EDEN group in five European countries illustrates the problem: A representative general population sample of 3,119 persons was patch tested with three TRUE Test panels, and a prevalence of positive patch test reactions (+, ++, +++) in the normal population of 25.2 % was observed. For metals in the standard series, this value was 15.4 %. When only those were considered who had a lifetime history of metal avoidance, this number decreased to 9.5 %. When it was additionally taken into consideration whether the volunteers had ever experienced contact dermatitis in their lifetime, only 3.6 % of the general population remained. This means that in 75 % of persons with positive patch test reactions to metals from the general population, these reactions are without relevance. In contrast, the proportion of relevant metal allergy in a cohort of eczema patients will be much higher as reported in many studies.

It is therefore wise to critically review the indication for patch testing in every patient, especially in referrals. While a study from the United Kingdom indicated that referrals to patch testing from GPs were generally appropriate [4], a more recent study from Italy indicated that a high proportion of referrals from GPs, ENT specialists, and even allergists for patch testing was not appropriate, resulting in a reduced sensitization rate [5].

Uncritical performance of patch testing, especially with known sensitizers such as paraphenylenediamine or acrylates, although not indicated, may unnecessarily induce active sensitization, although this is considered to happen rarely [6]. When a delayed patch test reaction is observed after 10 or more days, active sensitization should be suspected and confirmed by a repeated patch test of the substance, which then will be positive at 2–4 days [7].

A cause for possibly multiple false-positive patch test reactions ("excited skin syndrome," "angry back syndrome" [8]) may be the presence of active dermatitis. Thus, in patients with acute dermatitis, patch testing should be delayed until clearing of skin lesions.

False-negative reactions, on the contrary, may be due to any local or systemic immunosuppression. A frequent cause may be preceding intense exposure to natural or artificial UV irradiation. We therefore usually avoid patch testing in patients returning from a beach vacation or undergoing regular sunbathing or medical UV therapy. In this case, the patch test should be postponed by 4–6 weeks. Topical treatment with corticosteroids is well known to suppress patch test reactions, as is the systemic treatment with glucocorticosteroids, certainly if more than 20 mg of prednisone are taken daily [9]. A minimum of 7 days should be between discontinuation of topical corticosteroids and patch testing. No sufficient clinical data exist regarding the suppression of patch test reactions by topical immune modifiers and by oral immunosuppressants. We avoid patch testing in these situations unless an urgent indication exists. In mouse models, even more drugs were shown to suppress allergic contact dermatitis, such as calcium channel blockers, amiloride, pentoxifylline, pentamidine, clonidine, spiperone, N-acetylcysteine, and flavonoids [10]. The relevance of these findings to humans remains open. However, in our experience, there is no indication of a suppression of patch test reactions caused by the recently introduced systemic drug alitretinoin.

For legal purposes, we fully inform our patients about each diagnostic procedure including noninvasive ones such as patch testing and obtain informed consent. This should ideally be documented in writing. We therefore have developed a written informed consent form containing all information on the indication, benefits, and risks of patch testing to be signed before performance of the procedure.

3.3   Pitfalls in the Selection and Preparation of Allergens

Before patch testing can be performed, the appropriate patch test allergens have to be selected. While the standard series should always be tested, additional occupation or exposure-specific trays and allergens should be chosen based on history. The possible pitfalls can be to select too many irrelevant allergens, which may lead to an increase of false-positive reactions as described above on one side and the missing of important allergens with a high potential for relevance on the other side.

Patch test allergens should be of the highest possible quality. Therefore, if available, allergens from reliable commercial suppliers that are produced according to drug standards (good manufacturing practice) should be used. Indeed, in Germany, patch test allergens are regulated as drugs, which is not the case in many other countries. Allergen content in a patch test preparation may decay with time depending on environmental conditions. Therefore, the storage conditions and expiration dates prescribed by the manufacturer should be closely followed and monitored. A decay of allergen content due to improper storage conditions may occur, thus leading to false-negative reactions. Conversely, the oxidation of weak allergens may lead to highly sensitizing compounds [11].

Many allergens are not available as commercial test preparations and may have to be prepared by a pharmacy or the dermatologist's own laboratory. This leads to increasing complexity, with a potential for dilution errors resulting in possibly false-positive, false-negative, or irritant reactions. The same is true for the patch testing of the patient's own products that follow specific rules and cannot be treated here in detail. Recent reviews are available [12]. All dilution instructions should be documented in writing, and the documentation should be kept with patient data. It is often useful to test dilution series in patient's own products, e.g., in order to estimate the degree of concentration-dependent reactions.

In addition to patch test allergens, the quality of application systems should be considered. Chamber systems should provide sufficient and constant occlusion. Both aluminum and plastic-type chambers seem to fulfill these requirements. When testing fluids, differences in spreading were observed between both chamber types, leading to differentiated recommendations [13].

3.4 Pitfalls in the Application of Patch Test Allergens

Correct dispensing of patch test allergens is essential to achieve repeatable dosing [14–16]; otherwise, false-negative results may occur (Fig. 3.1). The whole test area has to be covered with the allergen in question, and spreading should be avoided. For Finn Chambers, 20 mg of petrolatum preparation seems to fulfill this requirement best [14]. Technicians should be well trained in dosing techniques, and training should be repeated in intervals.

Patch tests should be prepared shortly before application (maximum 2 h) to avoid oxidation or evaporation of allergens (especially fragrances) [17]. They should be placed on healthy, undamaged skin of the back in a well-documented and reproducible manner. In our department, we follow a standard application procedure and mark the tapes with a waterproof marker. In order to identify the patch test application sites, digital photos can be taken and stored; this is especially useful when late reactions are observed and no markings on the skin exist any longer.

The induction of an allergic delayed-type reaction depends on sufficient penetration of the allergen into the epidermis. Therefore, a complete occlusion during the application time should be achieved. Loosening of the patch test material and improper occlusion may lead to false-negative results. We therefore fixate the patches with a second layer of Fixomull (Beiersdorf, Germany). Profuse sweating in hot summer months, showering, and physical work or exercise may lead to loosening of the patches and impair patch test quality. Patients should be informed and abstain from exercise, physical work, and taking showers. Very hairy skin on the back is unsuitable for patch testing. It should be shaved first, but care has to be taken to avoid follicular irritant reactions. Usually, electric shaving is safer in this respect than wet shaving.

When a patch test to a substance that induced a strong reaction in the past is repeated, this patch should be placed a good distance from the next one to avoid spreading of the reaction and thus unreadability of the neighboring patches. If we deem such a repetition of a test to be warranted at all, we place the patch test usually on the upper arm a good distance from the other allergens. In case of intense and premature itching, patients may be instructed to return as early as 24 h after

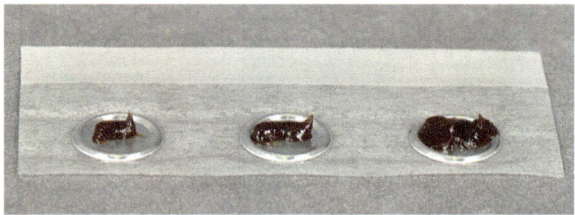

Fig. 3.1 Doses of petrolatum allergen preparations in Finn Chambers. Dosing Finn Chambers with 10 mg (*left*), 20 mg (*center*), and 40 mg (*right*) of a petrolatum allergen preparation; 20 mg is the correct dose. Doses that are too low may lead to unreliable or false-negative readings and doses that are too high, to spreading of the allergen

application in order to avert unnecessary intense reactions or even to pull off the patches themselves.

Testing in areas other than the back should be avoided, since patch test substances have been validated by testing on this skin. Other areas of the body may differ in penetration and irritation properties. If other patch test areas such as the upper legs have to be chosen, this should be well documented and taken into critical consideration.

Meteorological conditions at the time of patch testing may influence the results but only for weak reactions. A study of the German Contact Dermatitis Research Group indicated that with low temperature and humidity (i.e., winter conditions in Europe), both IR/? and + reactions were significantly increased with respect to the allergens fragrance mix, oil of turpentine, methyldibromo glutaronitrile + phenoxyethanol, and particularly formaldehyde, while ++/+++ reactions were hardly affected by weather conditions [18].

All nonstandardized patch test allergens, especially the patient's own substances as well as drugs, should be removed shortly after 20 min of application, and the test area should be inspected to avoid unanticipated toxic or immediate-type reactions followed by potential contact urticaria syndrome. Otherwise, the patch test has to remain on the skin for 24 or 48 h. Differences in exposure times were not shown to influence patch test results for standard allergens in a large study of the IVDK [19].

On removal of the patches, the patch test sites should be marked with a water-resistant pen. However, these may stain the underwear of patients. We mark the sites with tapes and use templates to locate individual patches.

3.5   Pitfalls in Reading and Interpreting the Patch Test Reaction

The reading of the patch test is in the center of the procedure and thus prone to many pitfalls. The basics are clear: Reading should follow the ICDRG guidelines [20, 21]. Optimal lighting is necessary, and in positive reactions, palpation is mandatory. The difficulties lie less in the grading of strong (++ and +++) reactions than in discriminating between doubtful (positive) and irritant reactions. Even experienced dermatologists were shown to differ in their readings, but consistency improved after a repetition of their patch test reading training [22]. This points at the need of recurrent training, especially if results are to be compared between centers. Excellent patch test reading training material can be accessed on the Internet (http://dkg.ivdk.org/).

It is important to read reactions consistently according to the morphology. Allergic reactions show erythema and infiltration covering the whole test area, possibly papules, vesicles, and bullae, and may spread beyond the patch test application site [22]. Doubtful reactions are defined as erythema and/or infiltration not covering the whole test area and few papules, but without erythema/infiltration covering the whole test area [22]. Irritant reactions are bullae, erosion, and dry or shiny skin, with possible cigarette paper structure, scaling, pustules, and petechiae. Some allergens, mostly disinfectants, preservatives, and emulgators (e.g., cocamidopropyl betaine), are notorious problem allergens known for frequently eliciting doubtful, weak, and false-positive test reactions [23]. Simultaneous sodium lauryl sulfate testing may help in the differentiation between allergic and irritant reactions [24]. However, even in the hands of the experienced, a repeated open application test may be necessary to confirm or rule out allergic contact dermatitis.

Another potential for pitfalls lies in the reading of skin-staining allergens such as povidone iodine (leaving a brown stain) that may be misinterpreted as erythema. Many pitfalls exist with the reading of reactions to patient's own substances. Mechanically irritating substances such as metal dust may cause follicular reactions, and false-positive patch tests may even be caused by microbial contamination of material [25].

Considering the skills and experiences needed for a correct reading of patch test reactions, this task should not be left to patients themselves. It has been shown that patients frequently misinterpret irritant patch test reactions as allergic (own unpublished data). If a patient is unable to return to the clinic for a reading due to any reason, we recommend at least to take a photo of the reaction(s) and to present it to us on the next appointment. Thereby, possibly necessary retesting can be confined to the number of allergens in questions.

Atypical, usually clearly irritant or even corrosive reactions should lead to reconsideration of the whole testing procedure, especially dilution steps in the testing of patient's own substances. In rare cases, dermatitis artefacta has to be taken into consideration [26]. Retesting with nonirritant patch test preparations (e.g., physiological saline) may clarify the situation.

A minimum of two readings, one 30 min after removal of the patch test and one a minimum of 24 h later, are obligatory not to miss any reactions, since positive reactions may develop later with some allergens (paraphenylenediamine, neomycin, bacitracin, corticosteroids, and blue disperse dyes) [27]. Furthermore, a decrescendo phenomenon on the second reading may reveal an irritant reaction, although this is not true in all cases [23]. There is no general agreement that late readings (days 6 or 7) should be performed on a regular basis, though it has been reported that additional information can be generated in a significant proportion of patients. Allergens most involved in producing late-positive reactions mentioned in the literature are nickel sulfate, neomycin sulfate, tixocortol-21-pivalate, p.t. butylphenol formaldehyde resin, Cl + Me isothiazolinone, and gold sodium thiosulfate [28, 29].

3.6   Pitfalls in Judging Patch Test Relevance

Every positive patch test reaction read as allergic should be judged regarding its clinical relevance. Relevance is defined as the capability of an information retrieval system to select and retrieve data appropriate to a patient's need [30]. In plain words, the information gained from patch testing should be useful for the patient to avoid sources of allergens leading to contact dermatitis in his private or occupational environment. Current relevance (CR) refers to the disease episode that leads the patient to the consultation and to subsequent patch testing. Past relevance (PR) refers to older clinical events that can be explained by the patch test data.

Judging of patch test relevance may be cumbersome. It involves a careful patient history, possibly additional testing procedures including patient's own products, information from manufacturers on the chemical composition of products, and, ideally, but frequently unavailable, a chemical analysis of products. Pitfalls exist in all the mentioned steps. The patient's memory may be unreliable, or he may have discarded products he used that lead to the clinical event. Product composition may have changed in the meantime without being communicated by manufacturers. Information from manufacturers regarding the composition of products may be unavailable or unreliable, especially if occupational substances are concerned. For cosmetics, the labeling of products is helpful, though not in all cases. In our experience, the best relevance judgments can be made in occupational cases when safety engineers of the occupational health insurance make actual workplace visits and take and analyze samples from the chemical environment.

For practical purposes, a simple relevance scoring system for positive patch test reactions has been proposed [30].

Practical Tips
- Only patch test patients with a positive history of dermatitis; otherwise, you will perform an epidemiological study and may see many difficult-to-interpret false-positive reactions.
- Be critical in patch testing with known sensitizers since you might actively sensitize a patient. There should be a history of contact to this substance.
- Avoid patch testing in the presence of active dermatitis. You might end up with an "angry back."
- Avoid patch testing after intensive UV exposure or under immunosuppression. Reactions may be false-negative.
- Test with high-quality allergens from reliable suppliers whenever possible.
- Always test with the standard series and choose additional allergens based on the history of the patient.
- If you test with a chamber system, make sure you use the correct allergen dose and that the patches remain well occluded.
- Be careful when retesting allergens that caused intense reactions in the past. You might see a spreading reaction or even generalized dermatitis.
- Reading of patch test reactions is an art. Follow the ICDRG guidelines and keep in good training.
- Perform a minimum of two readings; you might need even more.
- Do not forget to judge the relevance of a positive reaction and inform the patient about it.

References

 1. Wilf-Miron R, Lewenhoff I, Benyamini Z, Aviram A. From aviation to medicine: applying concepts of aviation safety to risk management in ambulatory care. Qual Saf Health Care. 2003;12(1):35–9.
 2. Moshell AN, Parikh PD, Oetgen WJ. Characteristics of medical professional liability claims against dermatologists: data from 2704 closed claims in a voluntary registry. J Am Acad Dermatol. 2012;66(1):78–85.
 3. Nethercott JR. Practical problems in the use of patch testing in the evaluation of patients with contact dermatitis. Curr Probl Dermatol. 1990;2(4):97–123.
 4. Lamb SR, Wilkinson SM. Audit of primary and secondary care as a source of patch test clinic referrals. Br J Dermatol. 2004;151(6):1258–60.
 5. Corazza M, Borghi A, Mantovani L, Virgili A. Analysis of patch test referrals: influence of appropriateness of referrals on sensitization rate. Contact Dermatitis. 2012;66(2):95–100.
 6. Devos SA, Van Der Valk PG. The risk of active sensitization to PPD. Contact Dermatitis. 2001; 44(5):273–5.
 7. Bruze M, Condé-Salazar L, Goossens A, Kanerva L, White IR. Thoughts on sensitizers in a standard patch test series. The European Society of Contact Dermatitis. Contact Dermatitis. 1999;41(5):241–50.
 8. Mitchell J, Maibach HI. Managing the excited skin syndrome: patch testing hyperirritable skin. Contact Dermatitis. 1997;37(5):193–9.
 9. Lindberg M, Matura M. Contact dermatitis. Heidelberg/New York: Springer; 2011.
10. Belsito DV. Patch testing with a standard allergen ("screening") tray: rewards and risks. Dermatol Ther. 2004;17(3):231–9.
11. Sköld M, Hagvall L, Karlberg A-T. Autoxidation of linalyl acetate, the main component of lavender oil, creates potent contact allergens. Contact Dermatitis. 2008;58(1):9–14.
12. Frosch PJ, Geier J, Uter W, Goossens A. Patch testing with the patients' own products. In: Contact dermatitis. Heidelberg/New York: Springer; 2011. p. 1107–19.
13. Isaksson M, Gruvberger B, Frick-Engfeldt M, Bruze M. Which test chambers should be used for acetone, ethanol, and water solutions when patch testing? Contact Dermatitis. 2007;57(2): 134–6.
14. Bruze M, Isaksson M, Gruvberger B, Frick-Engfeldt M. Recommendation of appropriate amounts of petrolatum preparation to be applied at patch testing. Contact Dermatitis. 2007; 56(5):281–5.
15. Bruze M, Frick-Engfeldt M, Gruvberger B, Isaksson M. Variation in the amount of petrolatum preparation applied at patch testing. Contact Dermatitis. 2007;56(1):38–42.
16. Frick-Engfeldt M, Gruvberger B, Isaksson M, Hauksson I, Pontén A, Bruze M. Comparison of three different techniques for application of water solutions to Finn Chambers®. Contact Dermatitis. 2010;63(5):284–8.
17. Gilpin SJ, Hui X, Maibach HI. Volatility of fragrance chemicals: patch testing implications. Dermatitis. 2009;20(4):200–7.
18. Uter W, Hegewald J, Kränke B, Schnuch A, Gefeller O, Pfahlberg A. The impact of meteorological conditions on patch test results with 12 standard series allergens (fragrances, biocides, topical ingredients). Br J Dermatol. 2008;158(4):734–9.
19. Brasch J, Geier J, Henseler T. Evaluation of patch test results by use of the reaction index. An analysis of data recorded by the Information Network of Departments of Dermatology (IVDK). Contact Dermatitis. 1995;33(6):375–80.
20. Maibach HI, Fregert S. Manual of contact dermatitis. Contact Dermatitis. 1980;6(7):430–4.
21. Fregert S. Manual of contact dermatitis: on behalf of the International Contact Dermatitis Research Group. Copenhagen: Munksgaard; 1974.
22. Svedman C, Isaksson M, Björk J, Mowitz M, Bruze M. 'Calibration' of our patch test reading technique is necessary. Contact Dermatitis. 2012;66(4):180–7.
23. Becker D. Allergic contact dermatitis. J Dtsch Dermatol Ges. 2013;11(7):607–21.

24. Löffler H, Becker D, Brasch J, Geier J, German Contact Dermatitis Research Group (DKG). Simultaneous sodium lauryl sulphate testing improves the diagnostic validity of allergic patch tests. Results from a prospective multicentre study of the German Contact Dermatitis Research Group (Deutsche Kontaktallergie-Gruppe, DKG). Br J Dermatol. 2005;152(4):709–19.
25. Schuster C, Mofarrah R, Aberer W, Kränke B. Pitfalls of patch testing with dental materials. Br J Dermatol. 2012;166(3):674–5.
26. Maurice PD, Rivers JK, Jones C, Cronin E. Dermatitis artefacta with artefact of patch tests. Clin Exp Dermatol. 1987;12(3):204–6.
27. Mowad CM. Patch testing: pitfalls and performance. Curr Opin Allergy Clin Immunol. 2006;6(5):340–4.
28. Davis MDP, Bhate K, Rohlinger AL, Farmer SA, Richardson DM, Weaver AL. Delayed patch test reading after 5 days: the Mayo Clinic experience. J Am Acad Dermatol. 2008;59(2): 225–33.
29. Jonker MJ, Bruynzeel DP. The outcome of an additional patch-test reading on days 6 or 7. Contact Dermatitis. 2000;42(6):330–5.
30. Lachapelle JM. A proposed relevance scoring system for positive allergic patch test reactions: practical implications and limitations. Contact Dermatitis. 1997;36(1):39–43.

The Validity of Patch Testing

4

Iris S. Ale

4.1 Introduction

Diagnostic tests are more or less objective methods that reduce the uncertainty factor in diagnosis. The validity of any test system represents its intrinsic ability to detect or measure the aimed biological phenomenon. A valid diagnostic test will supplement new information, allowing the clinician to make meaningful clinical inferences that lead to a change in management with a positive impact on the patient's outcome.

Patch testing is considered the most important diagnostic and investigative method currently available for studying allergic contact dermatitis (ACD) in clinical practice. The accurate diagnosis of the allergens responsible for the patient's dermatitis, through a properly performed and interpreted patch test, constitutes essential prerequisites for implementing adequate therapeutic and preventive measures. However, as a bioassay, patch testing still confronts several inherent methodological drawbacks and requires careful consideration of the technical aspects as well as critical assessment of the results. The issue of whether a positive patch test reaction is causally linked to the clinical dermatitis involves several pitfalls, including the inherent risk of false-positive and false-negative reactions and the difficulties in assessing clinical relevance. These issues are scarcely mentioned in the literature and are frequently overlooked in clinical studies.

4.2 Validating a Diagnostic Test

To validate a test as a diagnostic tool, we should be able to discriminate how many times the test has accurately categorized the tested subjects. In the case of patch testing, we must ascertain the test's ability to detect the existence of contact

I.S. Ale, MD
Department of Dermatology and Department of Allergy, School of Medicine,
Republic University of Uruguay, Arazati 1194 PC, Montevideo 11.300, Uruguay
e-mail: irisale@gmail.com

J.-M. Lachapelle et al. (eds.), *Patch Testing Tips*,
DOI 10.1007/978-3-642-45395-3_4, © Springer-Verlag Berlin Heidelberg 2014

Table 4.1 Patch testing outcomes

	Contact allergy		
Patch test result	**Present**	**Absent**	**Row total**
Positive	True positive (TP)	False positive (FP)	TP+FP Total number of subjects with a positive test
Negative	False negative (FN)	True negative (TN)	FN+TN Total number of subjects with a negative test
Column total	TP+FN Total number of subjects with contact allergy	FP+TN Total number of subjects without contact allergy	N=TP+TN+FP+FN Total number of subjects in the study

Key: True positive (TP)=number of patients with the disease who have a positive test result
True negative (TN)=number of patients without the disease who have a negative test result
False positive (FP)=number of patients without the disease who have a positive test result
False negative (FN)=number of patients with the disease who have a negative test result

sensitization to the tested substances. In other words, we have to establish the test's ability to detect both true-positive and true-negative reactions, while minimizing the number of false-positive and false-negative reactions. When considering the diagnostic utility of a test to identify persons with disease from persons without disease, reference is frequently made to common metrics, namely, *sensitivity*, *specificity*, *predictive value*, and *likelihood ratio*. These basic biostatistical concepts must be taken into consideration when validating a test as a diagnostic tool and are substantial in recognizing its inherent limitations. However, in reference to patch testing, they are rarely pondered in clinical studies or clinical diagnosis. Assessment of test performance is usually presented in a two-by-two contingency table that takes into account the screening test result (i.e., interpreted as positive or negative) and the presence or absence of the disease being studied (Table 4.1). Achieving this goal requires identifying beforehand which subjects had the disease being studied based on some reference test. The optimal design for assessing the validity of a diagnostic test is considered to be a prospective blind comparison of the test and a reference test or gold standard in a consecutive series of patients from a relevant clinical population [1]. As patch testing constitutes the only reliable test for diagnosis of contact allergy, the gold standard for comparison must be a confident clinical diagnosis made through the thorough study of each case and fulfillment of a precise case definition, in terms of the clinical findings, history of exposure, and reproducibility of the response with an appropriate time course after exposure [2]. Alternatively, a repeated open application test (ROAT) or a controlled exposure to the tested substance can be envisaged as a reference for comparison. However, these methods also have a certain degree of ambiguity and need further standardization [3, 4].

Originally, two-by-two tables were defined to analyze binary outcomes (two mutually exclusive categories such as death vs. survival, infected vs. noninfected) and their association with an equally dichotomous predictor variable (e.g., presence or absence of a pathogen). However, this is rarely the situation, since measurements of biological variables usually form a continuum of values. Continuous values can be made categorical by selecting a point (cutoff point) along the continuum and assigning all values on one side of that point to the abnormal category and those on the other side to the normal category. In such cases, the selection of a cutoff point to separate "positive" and "negative" results introduces a level of uncertainty, and there is almost always a certain degree of overlap between results from normal and diseased (abnormal) subjects. The choice of an appropriate cutoff has an important bearing on the calculated measures of test accuracy.

4.2.1 Sensitivity and Specificity

The key to patch testing is to allocate the tested individuals into either those who are allergic to the test chemical and should have a positive result or those who are not allergic, who should have a negative result. Those instances in which the test result is positive but no disease is present are called false-positive results. Conversely, the negative test results found when disease is actually present are called false-negative results. The proportion of subjects with a positive test result, of all those with disease, is known as the *sensitivity* of the test. In our scenario, it measures the proportion of allergic individuals that are correctly identified by the test; ergo, it represents the probability that a patch test result will be positive when contact allergy is present (true-positive rate) and is calculated using the formula: Sn = true positives/(true positives + false negatives). The higher the numerical value of sensitivity, the less likely the test returns false-positive results. Similarly, the proportion of subjects with a negative test result, of all those without contact allergy (true-negative rate), is known as the *specificity* of the test. It measures the proportion of individuals without contact allergy that are correctly identified by the test as nonallergic. Specificity is calculated using the formula: Sp = true negatives/(true negatives + false positives) (Table 4.2). Sensitivity and specificity are widely applied statistics used to quantify how good and consistent a test is. They provide stable estimates of the test's diagnostic discrimination and can be applied to any diagnostic test irrespective of the characteristics of the population on which the test is applied [5].

4.2.2 Predictive Values

Although the data about sensitivity and specificity are required to determine the validity and accuracy of a diagnostic test, from a clinical point of view, these indicators have a somewhat restricted usefulness. The major limitation of both sensitivity and specificity is that they are defined on the basis of people with or without a disease; therefore, they are of no practical use when it comes to helping the clinician estimate the probability of disease in individual patients. In clinical practice, it is more important to determine to what extent the test can help estimate the probability

Table 4.2 Sensitivity, specificity, and predictive values of patch test results

| | Contact allergy | | |
Patch test result	Present	Absent	Predictive value
Positive	True positive (TP)	False positive (FP)	Positive predictive value (TP/TP + FP)
Negative	False negative (FN)	True negative (TN)	Negative predictive value (TN/TN + FN)
	Sensitivity (TP/TP + FN)	**Specificity (TN/TN + FP)**	

Key: Sensitivity = TP/(TP + FN). Specificity = TN/(FP + TN). Positive predictive value = TP/(TP + FP). Negative predictive value = TN/(FN + TN). Positive likelihood ratio (LR+) = sensitivity/(1 − specificity). Negative likelihood ratio (LR−) = (1 − sensitivity)/specificity. Prevalence = (TP + FN)/(TP + FP + FN + TN). Pretest odds = prevalence/(1 − prevalence). Posttest odds = pretest odds × likelihood ratio. Posttest probability = posttest odds/(posttest odds + 1)

of the presence or absence of disease from an obtained test result—that is, how a particular test result predicts the risk of disease. There are two ways to quantify this inference: *predictive values* and *likelihood ratios*. Positive and negative predictive values describe a patient's probability of having (or not having) the disease once the results of his or her tests are known. The percentage of true-positive results out of all the positive test results is referred to as the positive predictive value (PPV) of the test (see Table 4.2). It represents the probability that a patient with a positive test result actually has the disease. Similarly, the percentage of true-negative results out of all the negative test results is referred to as the negative predictive value (NPV) of the test. The closer the PPV is to 100 %, the more likely the disease is present when the test is positive. If there were no false positives, the PPV would be TP/TP or 100 %. The closer the NPV is to 100 %, the more likely the disease is absent with a negative test finding. The PPV and NPV are of great importance for clinicians, who interpret the test results on a case-by-case basis. However, they not only depend on the test's properties but also on the prevalence of disease in the population. Therefore, they do not offer a single measure to describe the test's inherent accuracy. If the rate of contact allergy in the population tested is low, then the PPV decreases and the NPV increases. Conversely, when the rate of allergic persons tested increases (i.e., patch testing is used mostly to confirm the clinical diagnosis), then the PPV will increase at the same test sensitivity, whereas the NPV will decrease [6]. These statistical considerations have significant clinical implications. In clinical patch testing, positive reactions are at least ten times less frequent than negative ones. Therefore, even assuming that the test has high specificity, false-positive reactions will have a great impact on the proportion of true positives out of all positives elicited (i.e., the PPV of the test). This substantiates the importance of achieving a high prevalence rate of truly sensitized patients through a comprehensive clinical assessment before patch testing. Patch testing will be more cost-effective if there is a good pretest probability of ACD based on the comprehensive clinical evaluation and a careful selection of patients. Performing a patch test as a last diagnostic recourse in patients failing to meet the case definition for ACD will hardly be rewarding.

4.2.3   Likelihood Ratios and Diagnostic Odds Ratio

As the predictive values depend on the prevalence of the disease, they can rarely be generalized beyond a particular study (except when the study is based on a suitable random sample, as is sometimes the case for population screening studies). To remove the difficulty, decision analysts have suggested an alternative method to assess the predictive properties of a test: the likelihood ratio (LHR) [7–9]. LHRs are alternative statistics for summarizing the test's diagnostic accuracy, which are especially helpful in clinical practice. Conceptually, the LHR is the ratio of two probabilities, namely, the probability that a specific test result is obtained in patients with the disease divided by the probability of obtaining the same test result in patients without the disease. In the case of dichotomous test measures, the LHRs have a direct relationship with sensitivity and specificity that can be summarized as follows:

$$\text{Positive likelihood ratio}\left(\text{LHR}+\right) = \text{sensitivity}/\left(1-\text{specificity}\right)$$
$$\text{Negative likelihood ratio}\left(\text{LHR}-\right) = \left(1-\text{sensitivity}/\text{specificity}\right)$$

A LHR greater than 1 indicates that the test result is associated with the presence of the disease, whereas, an LHR lesser than 1 indicates that the test result is associated with the absence of disease. A LHR of 1 implies that the test result is equally likely to occur among patients with the disease as in patients without the disease.

The further LHR is from 1, the stronger the evidence for the presence or absence of the disease. LHRs above 10 and below 0.1 are considered to provide strong evidence to rule in or rule out diagnoses in most circumstances. LHR+from 5 to 10 and LHR- from 0.1 to 0.2 provide moderate evidence for the presence or absence of disease. Diagnostic tests with LHRs ranging from 0.33 to 3 rarely alter clinical decisions. LHRs are ratios of probabilities and can be treated in the same way as risk ratios for the purposes of calculating confidence intervals [9, 10]. Practically, LHRs may differ across various clinical settings and may be affected by the same limitations as predictive values. An alternative way to compare tests is by means of the diagnostic odds ratio. This indicator is calculated as the odds of a positive test result among those with the target condition divided by the odds of a positive test result among those without the condition and can be estimated as: (sensitivity × specificity)/[(1 − sensitivity) × (1 − specificity)] or as LHR+/LHR−

The values of OR range from zero to infinity, with higher values indicating better discriminatory test performance. Potentially helpful tests have diagnostic odds ratios higher than 20 [8].

4.2.4   Pretest and Posttest Probability

Clinical assessment begins with a preliminary clinical impression, a subjective pretest probability of disease. The ultimate goal of all diagnostic testing is to refine this pretest probability, allowing the physician to confirm or reject the initial diagnosis and make an informed treatment decision. All diagnostic tests will result in a change in the physician's probability of disease, the posttest probability. The degree to which a diagnostic test modifies the probability of disease from pretest to posttest represents the clinical utility of the test as measured by its operating characteristics. Useful tests generate changes from prior probability estimates to the posttest probability that alter treatment decisions and have a positive impact on the patient's outcome. Although patch testing is primarily conducted according to the clinical history and physical examination, it yields additional information that cannot be disclosed from the clinical history. Few studies have assessed the value of the clinical history and examination in the prediction of the test results and the incidence and relevance of clinically unsuspected positive patch tests [11–15].

Cronin [12] studied 1,000 patients by thorough clinical investigation and patch testing and demonstrated that the accuracy of the clinical prediction varies depending on the characteristics of the clinical dermatitis and the causative allergen. In a small group of patients having contact sensitization as the exclusive cause of their eczema (7 % of the total), the clinical anticipation of the patch test results was good (70 %). On the contrary, when the contact sensitization was incidental to the patient's primary dermatitis, the accuracy of clinical prediction was poor. Nickel was the most frequent sensitizer in women and the easiest to diagnose. Of the 84 nickel-sensitive women, the allergy was anticipated in 54 (64 %). Chromate, the commonest sensitizer in men, was suspected in only 40 % of the cases (19 out of 48). For other common allergens, such as lanolin and neomycin, sensitization was predicted in only 16 and 8 % of the cases, respectively. Similarly, Fleming et al. [13] demonstrated that clinical questions were accurate to predict the causative allergen in only 29–54 % of ACD cases, depending on the involved allergen. Reliable identification of causative allergens by history alone represents an overwhelming task in which we are usually unsuccessful. This is why patch testing is critical to the successful diagnosis of allergic contact dermatitis. Patch testing has been shown to be significant both in confirming contact sensitivities suspected from the clinical history and in unveiling unsuspected sensitivities. Podmore et al. [14] patch tested 100 consecutive patients; 41 of them were tested for screening purposes (e.g., eczema without an obvious allergic contact factor or clinical contact dermatitis without an obvious allergen). In 59 patients, a contact allergen was strongly suspected. Diagnosis was confirmed in 32 patients. In addition, 17 patients had 23 unexpected positive reactions. At least 50 % of the unexpected reactions were considered relevant to the patient's skin condition. If only the clinically suspected substances are tested, then all other possible sensitivities—which are not immediately evident from the history—would be neglected. For this reason, a standard series of allergens should be applied in all patients with suspected contact dermatitis. However, it must be remembered that a positive allergic patch test reaction only indicates that the subject has been previously exposed and sensitized to the tested allergen; it does not prove that the clinical exposure to the tested substance is the cause or an aggravating factor of the current dermatitis. Patch testing results require biological and clinical interpretation, and clinical relevance must be assessed for all positive reactions [15]. Although patch testing is primarily conducted according to the clinical history and physical examination, the diagnostic process is bidirectional, and test results will direct further questioning and investigation [16]. Reconsidering the history in light of the test results can lead to recognition of many hidden sources of causative exposure.

4.3 Validity of Patch Testing Results

Available data concerning validity of patch testing as a diagnostic tool are quite scarce because, on clinical grounds, we do not apply diagnostic tests to groups of subjects who are known to have the disease we are trying to diagnose (i.e., with definite contact sensitivity to the substances being tested). Likewise, data derived from testing in subjects without contact dermatitis are sparse. To assess the validity of patch test screening trays in the evaluation of patients with allergic contact dermatitis, Nethercott and Holness [17] tested 1,032 patients, 639 of them with the ICDRG standard series and 393 with the NACDG standard series. They found that sensitivity, specificity, positive accuracy, negative accuracy, and validity index for the ICDRG and NACDG screening series were 0.68, 0.77, 0.66, 0.79, and 0.72 and 0.77, 0.71, 0.66, 0.79, and 0.74, respectively. Using these estimates for sensitivity and specificity, we can calculate the LHR+: $= 0.68/(1-0.77) = 2.95$, and the LHR− $= (1-0.68)/0.77 = 0.43$. Therefore, although both screening series scored relatively high, nearly 30 % of all patch test results were considered inaccurate. Note, however, that the authors considered those patients with positive test results in which investigation did not provide evidence to support clinical relevance (either present or past) as having false-positive tests. Similarly, patients with negative test results to the screening series in which further testing revealed positive responses to other allergens were taken to have false-negative screening tests.

When assessing patch test validity, a major predicament derives from the fact that sensitivity, specificity, predictive values, or LHR data may be allergen-specific and will vary depending on the allergens tested and—to some extent—according to the score grading of the patch test reaction. Thus, we have to take into account that the accuracy of the clinical patch testing may be higher for one allergen than for another and, also, higher in strong positive reactions.

4.4 Issues That May Affect the Validity of Diagnostic Patch Testing

Conventional diagnostic patch testing has two main drawbacks: (1) it is very technique-dependent and (2) nonspecific reactions are more common than with other skin test methods. Standardization of the patch test materials and methodology is essential for attaining valid and reliable results. Significant research on chemical and toxicological aspects of test allergens, appropriate vehicles, and skin penetration has substantially contributed to the development of reliable and consistent patch test techniques. However, systematic studies for several important aspects of patch testing are lacking, and several sources of unreliability still exist, including

Table 4.3 Sources of unreliability in diagnostic patch testing

Materials
Different patch test systems
Different sources of patch test allergens
Different vehicles for allergens
Uneven distribution of allergens in the vehicle
Differences in concentration for some allergens
Degradation for some allergens
Testing nonstandardized allergens
Methodology
Variation in the amount of allergen applied
Variation in the skin occlusion and absorption
Differences in bioavailability and percutaneous penetration
Dissimilar pressure supported by the system according to the area of application
Different criteria of patient's selection
Application and reading times
Interpretation of the responses (intraindividual and interindividual variability)
Scoring scale applied
Technical
Partial or complete detachment of patches
Spillover due to excessive amount of allergen applied
Errors in the sequence of consecutive allergens
Biological
Unresponsiveness (overlooked intercurrent factors such as drugs, sun exposure, etc.)
Weak and doubtful responses
Summation of individual responses
Hyperresponsiveness and excited skin syndrome

variations in patch test materials, technique, and methodology, as well as inherent biological variability of patch test responses [18] (Table 4.3).

4.4.1 Issues Related to Allergen Characterization and Stability

Ideally, allergens should be well-defined chemical substances and have high purity and stability. Many allergens of the commercial patch test series are pure chemicals or chemically defined mixes of substances such as thiuram mix, fragrance mix, or caine mix. However, some testing materials are complex natural products, such as balsam of Peru, colophony, or wool alcohols. Much research is necessary to clarify the chemical structure of these natural materials and to define and characterize their allergenic fractions [19–24]. In addition, some studies have found poor stability for some allergens [25–27]. Allergenic degradation products can be formed during storage, mostly by auto-oxidation, as in the case of terpenes, such as limonene, geraniol, and linalool. In these circumstances, it may be difficult to determine the real allergenic fraction. The oxidized fragrance terpenes limonene, linalool, and linalyl acetate have been tested in consecutive dermatitis patients and demonstrated to be important contact allergens. From 2012, patch test preparations of oxidized limonene and oxidized linalool with defined content of the major allergens in the oxidation mixtures (i.e., the hydroperoxides) are commercially available [28–31].

4.4.2 Issues Related to Testing with Allergen Mixes

Allergen mixes were designed with the purpose of increasing the number of chemicals tested while decreasing the number of patches applied. Mixes are used as screening patch tests and, therefore, should have a high sensitivity. However, the use of mixes results in problems of concentration, interference, stability, formulation, and validation [32–47]. To prevent the occurrence of irritant reactions, the individual substances in the mix are frequently incorporated at suboptimal concentrations, which in turn may result in false-negative reactions. The fragrance mix I, introduced as a screening tool in the late 1970s by Larsen [36], contains eight fragrance materials: eugenol, isoeugenol, oak moss, geraniol, hydroxycitronellal, α-amylcinnamic aldehyde, cinnamic aldehyde, and cinnamic alcohol. It also contains the emulsifier sorbitan sesquioleate at 5 % in order to achieve a satisfactory dispersion of the constituents in the petrolatum vehicle. There have been discrepancies between the patch testing results with fragrance mix and its constituents. A positive reaction to one or more of the fragrance mix constituents is seen in only 40–70 % of patients with a positive reaction to fragrance mix [43–46]. Possible explanations for this inconsistency have been proposed by de Groot and Frosch [38], including (1) false-positive (irritant) reactions to the mix; (2) false-negative reactions to the constituents, which in turn may be due to (a) cross-reactions between chemically related substances in the mix, (b) an additive suprathreshold effect of the individual components in the mix, (c) enhancement in the absorption of the mix constituents by the emulsifier sorbitan sesquioleate (SSO), and (d) a marginally irritant constituent of the mix may enhance the absorption of other constituents; and (3) two or more constituents of the mix may form a new allergen ("compound allergy").

It has been suggested that the discrepancies between the results of testing with fragrance mix and its constituents were mostly due to the presence or absence of SSO [46]. The possibility of contact allergy to SSO has also been investigated. Contact dermatitis from sorbitol-based emulsifiers, commonly used in cosmetics and topical drugs such as topical corticosteroids, appears to be increasingly prevalent, and SSO has been considered an emerging allergen [48, 49]. In a multicenter European study, positive allergic reactions to SSO 20 % in petrolatum were observed in 0.7 % of the patients. The authors recommended the addition of SSO to the standard series in order to adequately evaluate a positive reaction to the fragrance mix [41]. Negative reactions to the mix with positive reactions to the ingredients also have been observed. De Groot et al. [39] tested 677 patients with fragrance mix I and its eight constituents. Sixty-one patients (9 %) reacted to the mix and to one or more of the ingredients, while 4 (0.6 of all patients and 6.2 % of all fragrance-sensitive patients) reacted to one of the individual ingredients in the absence of a reaction to the mix and were deemed to have false-negative reactions to the mix. Even if the proportion of false-negative results was low, given the high prevalence of fragrance allergy, the number of missed allergies with the currently used mix may attain clinical significance. Testing with the individual ingredients in those patients clinically suspected of having fragrance sensitivity but with a negative reaction to the mix may contribute to solve this problem. The same consideration is valid when there is a suspicion of a false-positive irritant reaction to the mix due to irritancy. Therefore, the currently used fragrance mix I (8 × 1 % with 5 % SSO) has been demonstrated to induce both false-negative [39, 40] and false-positive irritant reactions [41, 44] and leaves 20–30 % of fragrance sensitivities undetected.

To study the reliability of patch testing with mixes of rubber ingredients as a marker for the detection of contact allergy to any of its individual constituents, Geier and Gefeller [47] reviewed the results of 21,000 patients tested with mixes of rubber allergens, as well as the individual constituents. The gold standard for comparison was the breakdown patch testing, and the sensitivity of the mix was defined as the proportion of patients showing positive results to the mix among the number reacting to any of its single constituents. Of 222 patients with positive reactions to thiuram mix, 60 (27 %) did not react to any of the breakdown constituents and were deemed to have false-positive reactions to the mix. On the other hand, 32 (1.6 %) of the patients reacting to one or more of the individual constituents had a negative reaction to the mix and, therefore, were considered to have false-negative reactions. The statistics for thiuram mix were as follows: sensitivity of .84, specificity of .97, positive predictive value of .73, and negative predictive value of .98. For mercapto mix, the sensitivity was .57 and the specificity was .99; and for PPD black rubber mix, the sensitivity was .65 and the specificity was .99. The authors recommended breakdown testing for all positive reactions to the thiuram mix, as only about one-half of the patients positive to the mix had positive reactions to one of the individual components [47]. Mercapto mix and PPD black rubber mix demonstrated a low sensitivity. Chemical analyses on the stability of the mercapto mix components led to a new composition of the mix in 1995. In a subsequent study, Geier et al. observed that the combination of mercaptobenzothiazole (MBT) and mercapto mix had a sensitivity of 0.77 for detecting contact allergies to the MBT derivatives [50]. Therefore, they suggested to test both MBT and mercapto mix within the standard series.

4.4.3   Issues Related to the Vehicle of Patch Test Allergens

Choosing the appropriate vehicle for testing allergens is imperative for reliable patch testing. Vehicles influence bioavailability and percutaneous absorption of chemicals and may affect the reaction patterns of the allergens [51–60]. Petrolatum remains the standard vehicle for most allergens, with the exception of the TRUE Test. However, adequacy of petrolatum as a vehicle for many allergens has been questioned [55–60]. Patch test suspensions in petrolatum contain undispersed allergen particles, and both the particle size and number differ significantly between different test substances and different manufacturers [55, 56]. This phenomenon was specially described for metal salt preparations [57–60], and the nonhomogeneous release of allergen from the vehicle may result in false-positive reactions [59]. Other test substances, such as disperse dyes [61–63], also produced a number of problems. Ryberg et al. [61, 62]

analyzed commercial patch test preparations of eight different disperse dyes from different suppliers and observed wide variations in concentration compared with the label, impurities, and even presence of a different dye allergen in the final preparation. Frick et al. [63, 64] performed chemical analyses of 14 commercial test preparations of diphenylmethane −4,4'-diisocyanate in petrolatum and observed a poor correlation between the stated and found concentrations. Petrolatum patch test preparations are, for practical reasons, often placed in the test chambers in advance, several hours before the patient is tested. In this situation, some volatile patch test allergens evaporate from the preparations. Mowitz et al. [65] demonstrated that the concentration of four of the individual components of the fragrance mix I decreased by ≥20 % within 8 h when they were stored in Finn chambers at room temperature. When stored in a refrigerator, only the preparation of cinnamal had decreased by ≥20 % within 24 h [65]. Petrolatum samples of methyl methacrylate (MMA), 2-hydroxyethyl methacrylate (2-HEMA), 2-hydroxypropyl acrylate (2-HPA), cinnamal, and eugenol were stored in three different test chambers at room temperature and in a refrigerator. The decrease in concentration was substantial for all five allergens under both storage conditions for two of the chambers utilized [66]. Therefore, it has been recommended that the placement of the allergens in the test chambers should be done as closely as possible to the application of the test. Furthermore, storage in a refrigerator is recommended [65, 67]. Nowadays, advances are being made in the optimization of patch test preparations and the dispersion of allergens, and also the quality of these materials has significantly improved in the last 15 years [68], but not much significant research has been done on alternate vehicles in patch testing, and a universal optimal vehicle superior than petrolatum remains unfeasible [69]. Many of the abovementioned problems seem to be solved with the "ready to use" delivery systems, such as the TRUE Test, which has been pharmaceutically optimized concerning stability, solubility, and bioavailability of the allergens. The TRUE Test produces an exact dosage, even surface spread, and high bioavailability for the allergens. The allergen dosage has been determined by dose-response studies and the amount per unit area has been standardized [70, 71], solving the problems of low bioavailability, uncertain dosage, and uneven surface distribution, which are commonly seen when petrolatum is used as the vehicle. However, only the standard series and other additional allergens are currently available with the TRUE Test.

4.4.4 Issues Related to the Amount of Allergen Preparation Applied

Skin absorption can vary greatly depending on the patch test system used [72]. Factors such as conformity to the skin surface and degree of occlusion could be responsible for differences in the kinetics of allergen penetration. Variations in the amount of material applied can also lead to erroneous results. Excessive amounts can provoke spillover and irritant reactions, while inadequate dosing may, conversely, result in false-negative and doubtful reactions [73]. The ideal test situation is a test area completely covered with the test preparation without any spreading outside that area. The amount of material applied with the Finn

Chamber technique should be approximately 20 μL [74], but, as a manually dispensed system, the amount of allergen applied is potentially variable depending on technique [75, 76]. This variation was reported to be higher when testing allergens in solution [77].

4.4.5 Issues Related to the Allergen Concentration

The outcome of an individual patch test not only depends on the existence of delayed hypersensitivity to the tested substance but also on the test concentration, the application area, and the delivered dose, which, in turn, depend on the amount of percutaneous penetration induced by the method of exposure. Delayed sensitivity is a dose-related phenomenon, and there is a threshold surface concentration of allergen required to induce sensitization and/or elicitation of the response [78]. The concentration should be kept sufficiently high to detect contact hypersensitivity in weakly sensitized individuals but low enough to minimize the risk of false-positive irritant reactions. Almost any substance is capable of inducing irritant responses depending on the concentration and the method of exposure. When a test substance has low irritant properties, it is possible to use a relatively high elicitation threshold concentration; hence, allergic reactions will more likely be elicited. Correspondingly, if the substance has a fairly high irritancy potential, then a lower elicitation threshold concentration will have to be used to avoid the induction of false-positive irritant reactions. In the latter circumstance, allergic reactions are less likely elicited, especially in weakly sensitized persons; consequently, the risk of false-negative reactions will increase. Therefore, variations in the cutoff concentrations of the allergen will produce changes in the balance between positive and negative reactions [79–84]. If the elicitation threshold concentration is raised, both the true-positive and false-positive test results will increase and the number of false negatives will decrease; the sensitivity increases and specificity decreases. Conversely, if the elicitation threshold concentration is reduced, we will have fewer false-positive test results but also more false-negative responses. The specificity increases, but sensitivity declines. Therefore, the sensitivity and specificity of the test, as well as the predictive values, are related to the elicitation concentration.

The choice of allergen dose is frequently a delicate compromise; it should maximize the possibilities of obtaining true-positive results while minimizing the anticipated number of false-positive irritant results in nonallergic subjects. Commonly, patch test concentrations for many allergens, even for allergens in the recommended standard and screening trays, have been established in testing groups of patients supposed to have allergic contact dermatitis. In this context, a concentration is considered to be adequate when it is capable of eliciting a reasonable proportion of true-positive test results (i.e., positive results, which are accepted to be in association with the contact allergy to the test substance, based on clinical grounds) while eliciting a reasonably low proportion of irritant results according to morphological criteria. However, cutoff concentrations would be better estimated by employing the serial dilution test technique on patients proved to be sensitive to the tested substance, through controlled exposure, and, also, on nonsensitive controls. Using this technique, it would be possible to establish the concentrations eliciting strong, optimal, and minimal reactions. Thus, the mean standard error and ranges of reactivity for the different allergens can be calculated. Quantitative data about irritancy of the different substances can be obtained as well. This procedure has been used to standardize some patch testing materials, such as TRUE Test. The cutoff concentration for TRUE Test allergens was determined as the minimum concentration that caused a 2+ reaction in at least 90 % of the sensitive patients [35].

4.4.6 Issues Related to the Application of Multiple Patch Tests (Multi-testing)

With the premise of increasing the sensitivity of the patch test procedure and identify as many clinically relevant allergic subjects as possible, it is customary to utilize arrays of several allergens grouped as patch test series in the routine evaluation of patients with suspected ACD. When testing with allergen series, we are, in fact, performing several individual tests with different allergens. If the cutoff concentration for each individual allergen in the series was settled at a 95 % upper confidence limit, then, from a statistical viewpoint, each time we test 20 substances in a nonsensitized person, there would be a 100 % chance of eliciting a false-positive result from one of the substances tested. If we set the upper confidence interval at 99 % (i.e., assuming a false-positive response rate of only 1 % for each substance), we still have a 20 % possibility of eliciting a false-positive result each time we test 20 substances [85]. As we consider the tray of substances as a single screening test rather than an assemblage of individual substances, we are dealing with a confidence interval of 80 %, well below the conventional 95 % confidence interval used in other diagnostic tests. If we wish to use a 95 % confidence interval for patch test screening and reduce the number of false-positive reactions, it would be necessary to lower the cutoff concentration of the individual test substances, which will simultaneously reduce the true-positive response rate. Alternatively, we can consider reducing the number of chemicals tested to the indispensable minimum, selecting them carefully on the basis of the clinical history and exposure assessment. However, this measure would be detrimental, since it will diminish the screening capacity of the test and relevant allergies may be missed. All these concepts highlight the significance of carefully assessing the clinical relevance of all positive reactions. Diepgen and Coenraads [6] delineated another problem associated with testing multiple substances. When estimating differences in sensitization rates between two groups of subjects (e.g., between males and females or between atopics and nonatopics), we frequently perform pairwise comparisons using chi-square tests, one for each allergen tested, setting a p-value of 0.05 as statistically significant. In this circumstance, and for a series of only 10 allergens, there is a random possibility of over 40 % of finding by chance a statistically significant difference for at least one allergen between the two groups.

4.4.7   Issues Related to Patients' Selection

The validity of diagnostic patch testing depends largely on the clinical circumstances, especially on a good pretest probability based on careful patients' selection. To ensure a high PPV before patch testing, we should consider critically all the information about clinical history and physical exam and generate precise pretest probabilities of meeting the case definition for ACD. Patch testing is more effectively utilized as a confirming tool in those patients in which a diagnosis of ACD was made based on strict clinical criteria [16]. As we have already mentioned, testing patients failing to meet the case definition for ACD will hardly be cost-effective. However, if patch testing is performed in these patients, the practitioner should thoroughly assess the clinical relevance of all positive reactions. Another important issue refers to patch testing in populations. To determine sensitization rates in epidemiological studies, not only does the test system have to be well defined but even more so the test population. Sensitization rates in an insufficiently characterized test population can hardly reflect the number of clinically relevant sensitizations in the general population. Only data on clinically relevant sensitizations from a uniformly selected and well-characterized test population are suitable for making inferences. The pattern of allergic contact sensitization in a population is influenced by individual factors, such as sex, age, presence of atopy, presence of diseased skin, as well as factors related to exposure, including chemical structure of the allergen, concentration, climate, and industrialization [86]. An unequal frequency of positive patch tests is to be expected among groups of patients who differ with respect to individual variables. Christophersen et al. [87] evaluated the influence of individual factors on patch test results from consecutive patients in seven centers in Denmark during a 6-month period. They concluded that the results could only be compared after stratification or multivariate analysis and proposed a logistic regression model for standardization of the presentation of patch test results.

4.4.8   Issues Related to the Reading and the Interpretation of Patch Test Reactions

Even when the proposals of the International Contact Dermatitis Research Group in 1970 concerning a uniform terminology for patch test reading were generally accepted and represented a great advance [88] (Table 4.4), reading of patch test responses needs to be considered eminently subjective and constitutes one of the limitations of the method. Patch testing is a perceptual test, based on inspection and palpation of the test area. As any test that involves human perception and judgment, patch testing is bedeviled by variability of reporting on results. There are two forms of variability: (1) intra-observer variability (i.e., the phenomenon in which the same observer classifies the same test result differently on two separate occasions) and (2) interobserver variability (i.e., the phenomenon in which different observers classify the same test result differently). In epidemiological studies, this variability is recognized as an inevitable consequence of the use of perceptual tests. The classification

Table 4.4 Scoring of patch tests according to the International Contact Dermatitis Research Group (ICDRG)

Score	Reaction
– (0)	Negative reaction
?+	Doubtful reaction; erythema only
+ (1+)	Weak (nonvesicular) positive allergic reaction; erythema, infiltration, and possibly papules
++ (2+)	Strong (vesicular) positive allergic reaction; erythema, infiltration, papules, and vesicles
+++ (3+)	Extreme positive allergic reaction; bullous reaction
IR	Irritant reaction

and score grading of patch test reactions depend on descriptive morphology. Typical morphological features of an allergic test response are erythema, edema, papules, and vesicles (or bullae). The significant point in assessing a positive patch test response is ascertaining whether it represents an allergic reaction or a false-positive reaction. At least an erythematous infiltration should be present for a reaction to be considered allergic, while reactions that show only erythema without infiltration—called doubtful reactions—are frequently nonspecific or correspond to irritancy. Allergic patch test reactions are traditionally scored in terms of intensity, and a grading scale from 1+ to 3+ is now generally accepted for ranking these allergic reactions. Even when all reading systems are based on the same morphological features, there remains some variation in the exact definition of the different grades of this scale between the different working groups. For instance, there are discrepancies in the reading of the 1+ reaction between the different contact dermatitis groups. It has been proposed [89] to introduce an extra grade of patch test reaction in the scoring and distinguish between 1(+) reaction, characterized by homogeneous redness in the test area with scattered papules, and 2(+) reaction, characterized by homogeneous redness and homogeneous infiltration in the test area. However, it is debatable whether this distinction may have practical benefits. In contrast, other authors have suggested that a simplified score may reduce the interindividual variations in patch test readings [90]. No real consensus has been reached in this matter so far. Such minor differences of categorization may determine variations in interpretation of the responses. Bruze et al. [91] studied the accordance in patch test readings and showed that there is good accordance among various readers, except with the NACDG system. The morphological feature that seemed most difficult to evaluate was the papule, so perhaps it would be convenient not to demand the existence of this feature as essential for the categorization of a patch test reaction as allergic.

Concerning the application time, routine patch testing is usually performed with 48-h occlusion. However, some centers prefer 24-h occlusion. A comparative study using simultaneous duplicate TRUE Test standard series in 250 consecutive patients and removing one series after 24 and the other after 48 h demonstrated a high overall concordance of results. However, it was also observed that clinically relevant allergens would have been missed in 16 patients if only the 24-h occlusion test was performed [92].

The time of reading has been standardized [93] but is somewhat variable between different patch test clinics. Usually, the first reading is performed at day 2 (48 h) after patch test application, approximately 30 min after taking off the patches, and the second reading is performed at 72 or 96 h after application. Unfortunately, the timing of the reactions to different allergens does not necessarily follow the timing of the readings. Delayed readings, 1 week after application, are highly recommended, especially for some slow-reacting allergens, such as neomycin or corticosteroids, among others; even nickel may behave as a slow-reacting allergen [93–96]. Patch test results should be read at least in two successive opportunities, without which their accuracy is seriously impaired. A single reading on day 2 (48 h) may determine that approximately 30 % of the contact allergies detected by the standard series are missed, as compared with the number of allergies found when the test is read repeatedly up until 1 week from patch test application [93]. In addition, multiple readings are crucial in distinguishing false-positive reactions. However, if only one reading is feasible, it should be performed on day 3 or 4 [93]. Doubtful and weak reactions require a cautious interpretation and a careful consideration of the clinical circumstance. When a weak reaction correlates with the clinical picture, it may be significant [97]. Because of biological or technical reasons, there might be a variation in the intensity of the test response to the same allergen from time to time. To establish or rule out contact allergy, merely repeating the patch test may be sufficient to demonstrate that a doubtful or weak reaction is not consistently obtainable and, therefore, likely represents a false-positive reaction. If required, patch test concentration may be raised and/or additional tests such as intradermal testing or provocative testing may be performed.

4.4.9 The Problem of False-Positive and False-Negative Patch Test Reactions

The ideal patch test should correctly diagnose contact sensitization detecting both true-positive and true-negative reactions while minimizing the number of false-positive and false-negative reactions. However, even when an appropriate testing technique is applied, false-negative and false-positive reactions may occur. The background of false-positive test reactions is usually irritancy. Although the recommended test concentration for the sensitizers in the standard series is the result of extensive international experience on testing, some of the concentrations (e.g., for chromate, epoxy resin, and formaldehyde) have been chosen too close to the irritancy threshold in order to diminish the risk of obtaining false-negative reactions. A false-positive reaction may be attributed to several causes, such as (1) testing with allergens that are marginally irritants, (2) testing with allergens at concentrations that exceed their irritancy thresholds, (3) spillover reaction from a nearby true positive reaction, (4) multiple simultaneous positive reactions, (5) testing patients with active dermatitis or otherwise sensible or irritable skin, and (6) testing with nonstandardized substances or substances of unknown irritant potential. Certainly, this list is not exhaustive. Irritant reactions are often morphologically indistinguishable from allergic ones. Especially, weak allergic reactions can be clinically indistinguishable from false-positive reactions. The distinction is not necessarily provided by conventional histology, nor yet appropriately resolved by specialized immunologic [98] or bioengineering techniques [99–102]. Reaction dynamics can be integrated into the assessment of test reactions as allergenic or irritant: A crescendo pattern (increase in reaction severity between the 24/48-h and 72-h readings) or a "plateau" reaction (consistent reaction severity) tends to suggest a genuine allergic reaction, while a "decrescendo" pattern (decrease in reaction severity between the 24/48-h and 72-h readings) suggests irritation. We must remember that the threshold for irritancy shows huge variance among individuals. Testing with the nonallergenic obligatory irritant aqueous sodium lauryl sulfate (SLS) 0.25 %, performed in parallel with patch testing with allergenic preparations, provides information on the irritability of the skin at the time of testing and facilitates the evaluation of doubtful and weak reactions. The open use or provocative test may sometimes distinguish an allergic from an irritant response, because open testing is far less likely than closed testing to produce an irritant reaction. Ideally, the ambivalent patch test should be repeated, preferably incorporating a dose-response assessment (serial dilution) [103].

The frequency of false-negative reactions is difficult to evaluate. Even with appropriate patch test material, there may be several reasons for false negativity, most often insufficient penetration of the allergen. A false-negative reaction can occur for a number of reasons: (1) failure to perform delayed readings, which is especially important for allergens known to elicit delayed reactions, and when testing elderly patients, who may present a protracted immunologic response; (2) the test concentration and/or the amount of the substance applied may have been insufficient; (3) the vehicle may not have released a sufficient amount of the allergen (the biological availability was too low); (4) the patient's skin was unresponsive by prior sun exposure, local application of corticosteroids, and systemic administration of corticosteroids or immunosuppressors or other causes of skin hyporeactivity [104]; (5) the test site might have been inappropriate; (6) the occlusion might have been inadequate; and (7) there was an unsatisfactory replication by the test of the real exposure conditions (e.g., occlusion, heat, mechanical trauma, etc., that might enhance the percutaneous penetration of the allergens) or the skin penetration at the test site is lower than that of clinical exposure (e.g., eyelids, axillae, etc.). When patch testing with a particular substance is negative in a patient suspected to have a dermatitis from contact with that substance, the putative allergen should be retested—perhaps in a different concentration, with a different vehicle, or with a different testing method, such as the ROAT.

4.4.10 The Problem of Patch Test Reproducibility

The value of any test depends on its ability to yield the same result when reapplied to stable patients. Reproducibility of patch testing, defined as the test's ability to give consistent results when testing is repeatedly performed on the same individual, has been frequently questioned.

Gollhausen et al. [105] double-tested concomitantly on the left and right sides of the upper back 35 patients with allergens from the standard series and some vehicles (ointments) and found that 43.8 % of the positive allergic reactions were non-reproducible. In a multicenter study from the German Contact Dermatitis Research Group [106], 1,285 patients were double-tested concomitantly with 10 allergens from the standard series and manually loaded patch test systems. Non-reproducible allergic reactions were seen in 194 patients (15.1 %). The authors concluded that non-reproducibility was allergen-dependent. The likelihood of non-reproducible allergic reactions increased when more than four positive reactions were seen at the same time and with another positive reaction located in close proximity to an allergic reaction. Other authors reported a high reproducibility for concomitant patch test reactions. Lindelöf [107], testing 220 consecutive patients, obtained a nonreproducibility rate of 9.5 %, Bousema et al. [108] obtained 93 % of concordant allergic results, and Bourke et al. [109] reported 8 % of completely discordant results and observed that many non-reproducible results were not relevant. Some of the variability is eliminated by the use of ready-to-use patch test systems. Lachapelle [110] tested 100 consecutive patients, using Epiquick, and observed a non-reproducibility rate of only 4.2 %. Ale and Maibach [111], using TRUE Test in 500 consecutive patients, obtained 95 % of concordant allergic results. Therefore, it appears that the differences in the reproducibility of patch testing are mainly due to methodological aspects.

4.4.11 Issues Related to the Assessment of Clinical Relevance

Patch testing results require biological and clinical interpretation. The fact that contact allergy to certain allergen(s) has been reliably demonstrated by careful patch testing does not prove that such allergen(s) is responsible for the patient's ACD. A true-positive patch test reaction only indicates that the patient has been previously exposed and sensitized to the substance. Patients may suffer major changes in their lifestyle on the basis of patch testing results; therefore, it is crucial to establish that the positive reaction is actually linked to the clinical dermatitis, either as a primary cause or as an aggravating factor. Assessing the relevance of a positive patch test reaction is complex and involves many confounding factors. According to the well-established criteria [112], we consider that a positive patch test reaction is "relevant" if the allergen is traced. If the source of a positive patch test is not traced, we consider it as an "unexplained positive." We use "current" or "present" relevance if the positive patch test putatively explains the patient's present dermatitis. Likewise, when the positive patch test explains a past clinical disease not directly related to the current symptoms, we refer to this as "past" relevance. However, recurrent but discontinuous contact with an allergen can occur in some patients, providing difficulty in discriminate between current and past relevance. From a practical perspective, establishing that a positive reaction has past relevance or possible relevance does not direct the clinician to intervene directly for the very problem for which past testing was performed. However, reporting not currently relevant data serves an important epidemiological role and may be useful in preventing further outbreaks of ACD in a patient. The determination of relevance primarily depends on the expertise of the investigator and the possibility of detecting the allergen in the environment of the patient. Guidelines for assessment of relevance have been proposed [113]. Relevance scores and accuracy of the assessment are significantly improved by a comprehensive knowledge of the patient's chemical environment. Often, a visit to the patient's workplace proves rewarding. Besides patch testing, other types of skin tests, such as open and semi-open tests, tests with product extracts, and ROAT, may be required to establish a definite causative relationship between the positive patch test result and the clinical dermatitis. The ROAT has significant potential in refinement of the evidence-based diagnosis of clinical relevance. This test is not standardized to the same extent, and it is time-consuming, but mimics some real-life exposure situations. However, for general validation, a standardized measurement of the results of ROAT, such as the ICDRG scoring system for patch testing, is required [3].

Conclusion

The outlined evidence suggests that, even if patch testing has limitations from the standpoint of its validity, it can be effectively used as a diagnostic test to establish the presence of contact sensitization to the test chemicals. The allergens in the standard series recommended by the ICDRG, EEGDRG, and NACDG are most likely to disclose valid and reliable results. However, several aspects of the patch test procedure should be considered to reduce the risk of spurious false-positive or false-negative responses. The strategy for maximizing the efficacy and accuracy of patch testing includes the adoption of strict criteria for the selection of patients, further standardization of the patch technique, improved use of dose-response assessments, and, above all, refined and rigorous procedures for the assessment of clinical relevance of the patch test reactions. Patients may suffer major changes in their lifestyle on the basis of patch testing results; therefore, it is crucial to establish that the positive reaction is actually linked to the clinical dermatitis. Patch testing may furnish information that cannot be disclosed from the clinical history and usually proves essential to the adequate treatment and prevention of recurrence. Providing an objective proof of the allergic condition, patch testing is essential for patient cooperation in allergen avoidance. Recent decades have provided many advances, but much remains to be done.

Practical Tips
- Use strict criteria for the selection of patients to generate high pretest probabilities of contact sensitization.
- Always start with a complete clinical history and a careful physical examination.
- Make an effort to adopt a meticulous patch testing technique and methodology.

- The amount of allergen placed in the chamber should cover the test area completely, without any spreading outside that area, to prevent overlapping at reading.
- The amount of allergen placed in the different chambers should be as uniform as possible.
- The placement of the allergens in the test chambers should be done as closely as possible to the application of the test.
- The allergens supplied in aqueous solutions should be applied immediately before applying the test to avoid evaporation of liquids.
- Avoid testing with test materials degraded by poor storage or aging.
- Avoid testing with poorly characterized test materials.
- Readings should be done at least in two successive opportunities (conventionally, 20–30 min after the removal of the patches and also after 96 or 72 h).
- Late readings, 7 days after patch test application are highly recommended.
- Make efforts to avoid false-positive or false-negative patch test reactions.
- Avoid testing patients with active dermatitis.
- Unless inevitable, avoid testing patients in treatment with corticosteroids or immunosuppressors or otherwise hyporeactive skin.
- Test with the obligatory irritant SLS 0.25 %, in parallel with patch testing to reveal an eventual irritability of the skin at the time of testing.
- Avoid occlusive testing with substances of unknown irritant potential.
- When using nonstandardized allergens, select appropriate concentrations and vehicles and/or perform open or semi-open test and/or perform tests in control subjects.
- The presence of many positive reactions and/or unusually strong reactions should raise awareness of a hyperirritable state.
- Retest the responsible allergen using serial dilution.
- Perform ROAT or provocative use testing (PUT).
- Always determine the clinical relevance of the positive patch test reactions.
- Seek for sources of relevant exposure.
- Consider cross-reacting substances.
- Consider concomitant and simultaneous sensitization.
- Consider indirect, accidental, or seasonal contact.
- Obtain information about environmental allergens from databases, product labeling, material safety data sheets, textbooks, etc.
- Obtain information from the product's manufacturer.
- Perform chemical analysis of products.
- Perform exposure assessment.
- When in doubt and especially in doubtful or weak (+) positive reactions, additional complementary testing approaches should be implemented.
- Repeat patch testing to confirm its reproducibility.

- Perform patch testing using a range of concentrations (dose-response assessment) and/or a different vehicle.
- Perform patch testing using chemically related substances.
- Perform patch testing with products containing the suspected allergen and/or product extracts.
- Perform open or semi-open tests, ROAT, and PUT.

References

1. Lijmer JG, Willem Mol B, Heisterkamp S, Bonsel GJ, Prins MH, van der Meulen JH, et al. Empirical evidence of design-related bias in studies of diagnostics tests. JAMA. 1999;282:1061–6.
2. Ale SI, Maibach HI. Operational definition of allergic contact dermatitis. In: Maibach H, editor. Toxicology of skin. Philadelphia: Taylor & Francis; 2001. p. 345–55.
3. Nakada T, Hostynek JJ, Maibach HI. Use tests: ROAT (repeated open application test)/PUT (provocative use test) an overview. Contact Dermatitis. 2000;43:1–3.
4. Johansen JD, Bruze M, Andersen KE, Frosch PJ, Dreier B, White IR, et al. The repeated open application test: suggestions for a scale of evaluation. Contact Dermatitis. 1997;39:95–6.
5. Nethercott J. Sensitivity and specificity of patch tests. Am J Contact Dermat. 1994;5:136–42.
6. Diepgen TL, Coenraads PJ. Sensitivity, specificity and positive predictive value of patch testing: the more you test, the more you get? Contact Dermatitis. 2000;42:315–7.
7. Slawson DC, Shaughnessy AF. Teaching information mastery: the case of Baby Jeff and the importance of Bayes' theorem. Fam Med. 2002;34:140–2.
8. Deeks JJ, Altman DG. Diagnostic tests 4: likelihood ratios. Br Med J. 2004;329:168–9.
9. Dujardin B, Van den Ende J, Van Gompel A, Unger JP, Van der Stuyft P. Likelihood ratios: a real improvement for clinical decision making? Eur J Epidemiol. 1994;10:29–36.
10. Pauker SG, Kassirer JP. The threshold approach to clinical decision making. N Engl J Med. 1980;302:1109–17.
11. Agrup G, Dahlquist I, Fregert S, Rorsman H. Value of history and testing in suspected contact dermatitis. Arch Dermatol. 1970;101:212–5.
12. Cronin E. Clinical prediction of patch test results. Trans St John's Hosp Derm Soc. 1972;58:153–62.
13. Fleming CJ, Burden AD, Forsyth A. Accuracy of questions related to allergic contact dermatitis. Am J Contact Dermat. 2000;11:218–21.
14. Podmore P, Burrows D, Bingham EA. Prediction of patch test results. Contact Dermatitis. 1984;11:283–4.
15. Ale SI, Maibach HI. Clinical relevance in allergic contact dermatitis, an algorithmic approach. Dermatosen. 1995;43:119–21.
16. Ale SI, Maibach HI. Diagnostic approach in allergic and irritant contact dermatitis. Expert Rev Clin Immunol. 2010;6(2):291–310.
17. Nethercott JR, Holness L. Validity of patch test screening trays in the evaluation of patients with allergic contact dermatitis. J Am Acad Dermatol. 1989;21:568.
18. Fischer TI, Hansen J, Kreilgård B, Maibach HI. The science of patch test standardization. Immunol Allergy Clin. 1989;9:417–34.
19. Karlberg AT. Contact allergy to colophony. Chemical identifications of allergens, sensitization experiments and clinical experiences. Acta Derm Venereol Suppl (Stockh). 1988;139:1–43.

20. Karlberg AT, Lidén C. Comparison of colophony patch test preparations. Contact Dermatitis. 1988;18:158–61.
21. Karlberg AT, Lidén C. Clinical experience and patch testing using colophony (rosin) from different sources. Br J Dermatol. 1985;113(4):475–81.
22. Mitchell JC. Patch testing with some components of balsam of Peru. Contact Dermatitis. 1975;1(6):391–2.
23. Matthies C, Dooms-Goossens A, Lachapelle JM, Lahti A, Menné T, White IR, et al. Patch testing with fractionated balsam of Peru. Contact Dermatitis. 1988;19:384–9.
24. Hausen BM. Contact allergy to balsam of Peru. II. Patch test results in 102 patients with selected balsam of Peru constituents. Am J Contact Dermat. 2001;12(2):93–102.
25. Nilsson U, Magnusson K, Karlberg O, Karlberg AT. Are contact allergens stable in patch test preparations? Investigation of the degradation of d-limonene hydroperoxides in petrolatum. Contact Dermatitis. 1999;40:127–32.
26. Erikstam U, Bruze M, Goossens A. Degradation of triglycidyl isocyanurate as a cause of false-negative patch test reaction. Contact Dermatitis. 2001;44:13–7.
27. Sadhra S, Foulds IS, Gray CN. Oxidation of resin acids in colophony (rosin) and its implications for patch testing. Contact Dermatitis. 1998;39:58–63.
28. Karlberg AT, Dooms-Goossens A. Contact allergy to oxidized d-limonene among dermatitis patients. Contact Dermatitis. 1997;36:201–6.
29. Matura M, Goossens A, Bordalo O, Garcia-Bravo B, Magnusson K, Wrangsjo K, et al. Oxidized citrus oil (R-limonene): a frequent skin sensitizer in Europe. J Am Acad Dermatol. 2002;47:709–14.
30. Matura M, Goossens A, Bordalo O, Garcia-Bravo B, Magnusson K, Wrangsjo K, et al. Patch testing with oxidized R-(+)-limonene and its hydroperoxide fraction. Contact Dermatitis. 2003;49:15–21.
31. Matura M, Skold M, Borje A, Andersen KE, Bruze M, Frosch P, et al. Selected oxidized fragrance terpenes are common contact allergens. Contact Dermatitis. 2005;52:320–8.
32. Mitchell JC. Patch testing with mixes. Note on mercaptobenzothiazole mix. Contact Dermatitis. 1981;7:98. 68, 70, 76, 77.
33. Lynde CW, Mitchell JC, Adams RM, Maibach HI, Schorr WJ, Storrs FJ, et al. Patch testing with mercaptobenzothiazole and mercapto-mixes. Contact Dermatitis. 1982;8:273–4.
34. Menne T, Hjorth N. Routine patch testing with paraben esters. Contact Dermatitis. 1988;19:189–91.
35. Kreigård B, Hansen J, Fischer T. Chemical, pharmaceutical and clinical standardization of the TRUE Test caine mix. Contact Dermatitis. 1989;21:23–7.
36. Larsen WG. Allergic contact dermatitis to the perfume in Mycolog cream. J Am Acad Dermatol. 1979;1:131–3.
37. Larsen WG. Perfume dermatitis. J Am Acad Dermatol. 1985;12:1–9.
38. de Groot AC, Frosch PJ. Adverse reactions to fragrances. Contact Dermatitis. 1997;36:57–86.
39. de Groot AC, van der Kley AM, Bruynzeel DP, Meinardi MM, Smeenk G, van Joost T, et al. Frequency of false-negative reactions to the fragrance mix. Contact Dermatitis. 1993;28:139–40.
40. Frosch PJ, Pilz B, Andersen KE, Burrows D, Camarasa JG, Dooms-Goossens A, et al. Patch testing with fragrances: results of a multicenter study of the European Environmental and Contact Dermatitis Research Group with 48 frequently used constituents of perfumes. Contact Dermatitis. 1995;33(5):333–42.
41. Frosch PJ, Pilz B, Burrows D, Camarasa JG, Lachapelle JM, Lahti A, et al. Testing with the fragrance mix – is the addition of sorbitan sesquioleate to the constituents useful? Contact Dermatitis. 1995;32(5):266–72.
42. Larsen W, Nakayama H, Fischer T, Elsner P, Frosch P, Burrows D, et al. A study of new fragrance mixtures. Am J Contact Dermat. 1998;9:202–6.
43. Malanin G, Ohela K. Allergic reactions to fragrance mix and its components. Contact Dermatitis. 1989;21:62–3.

44. Enders F, Przybilla B, Ring J. Patch testing with fragrance mix at 16 % and 8 %, and its individual constituents. Contact Dermatitis. 1989;20:237–8.
45. Johansen JD, Menné T. The fragrance mix and its constituents: a 14-year material. Contact Dermatitis. 1995;32:18–23.
46. Enders F, Przybilla B, Ring J. Patch testing with fragrance mix and its constituents. discrepancies are largely due to the presence of sorbitan sesquioleate. Contact Dermatitis. 1991;24:238–9.
47. Geier J, Gefeller O. Sensitivity of patch tests with rubber mixes: Results of the Information Network for Departments of Dermatology from 1990 to 1993. Am J Contact Dermat. 1995;6:143–9.
48. Asarch A, Scheinman PL. Sorbitan sesquioleate: an emerging contact allergen. Dermatitis. 2008;19(6):339–41.
49. Orton DI, Shaw S. Sorbitan sesquioleate as an allergen. Contact Dermatitis. 2001; 44(3):190–1.
50. Geier J, Uter W, Schnuch A, Brasch J. Diagnostic screening for contact allergy to mercaptobenzothiazole derivatives. Am J Contact Dermat. 2002;13(2):66–70.
51. Tanglertsampan C, Maibach HI. The role of vehicles in diagnostic patch testing. A reappraisal. Contact Dermatitis. 1993;29:169–74.
52. Marzulli FN, Maibach HI. Effect of vehicles and elicitation concentration in contact dermatitis testing (I). Experimental contact sensitization in humans. Contact Dermatitis. 1976; 2:325–9.
53. Marzulli FN, Maibach HI. Further studies of the effects of vehicles and the elicitation concentration in experimental contact sensitization testing in humans. Contact Dermatitis. 1980;6:131–3.
54. Atkinson JC, Rodi SB. Effects of vehicles and elicitation concentration in contact dermatitis testing. II. Statistical analysis of data. Contact Dermatitis. 1976;2:330–4.
55. Fischer T, Maibach HI. Patch test allergens in petrolatum: a reappraisal. Contact Dermatitis. 1984;11:224–8.
56. Vanneste D, Martin P, Lachapelle J-M. Comparative study of the density of particles in suspensions for patch testing. Contact Dermatitis. 1980;6:197–203.
57. Wahlberg JE. Petrolatum-A reliable vehicle for metal allergens? Contact Dermatitis. 1980;6:134–6.
58. Van Ketel WG. Petrolatum again: an adequate vehicle in cases of metal allergy? Contact Dermatitis. 1979;5:192–3.
59. Fisher T, Rystedt I. False-positive, follicular and irritant patch test reactions to metal salts. Contact Dermatitis. 1985;12:93–8.
60. Skog E, Wahlberg JE. Patch testing with potassium dichromate in different vehicles. Arch Dermatol. 1969;99:697–700.
61. Ryberg K, Gruvberger B, Zimerson E, Isaksson M, Persson L, Sörensen O, et al. Chemical investigations of disperse dyes in patch test preparations. Contact Dermatitis. 2008;58:199–209.
62. Ryberg K, Goossens A, Isaksson M, Gruvberger B, Zimerson E, Persson L, et al. Patch testing of patients allergic to Disperse Blue 106 and Disperse Blue 124 with thin-layer chromatograms and purified dyes. Contact Dermatitis. 2009;60:270–8.
63. Frick-Engfeldt M, Zimerson E, Karlsson D, Skarping G, Isaksson M, Bruze M. Is it possible to improve the patch-test diagnostics for isocyanates? A stability study of petrolatum preparations of diphenylmethane-4,4′-diisocyanate and polymeric diphenylmethane diisocyanate. Contact Dermatitis. 2007;56(1):27–34.
64. Frick-Engfeldt M, Isaksson M, Zimerson E, Bruze M. How to optimize patch testing with diphenylmethane diisocyanate. Contact Dermatitis. 2007;57(3):138–51.
65. Mowitz M, Zimerson E, Svedman C, Bruze M. Stability of fragrance patch test preparations applied in test chambers. Br J Dermatol. 2012;167(4):822–7.
66. Mose KF, Klaus E, Andersen KE, Christensen LP. Stability of selected volatile contact allergens in different patch test chambers under different storage conditions. Contact Dermatitis. 2012;66:172–9.

67. Buckley DA. Advance preparation of some patch test series should be avoided. Br J Dermatol. 2012;167(4):708–9.
68. Nakada T, Hostýnek JJ, Maibach HI. Nickel content of standard patch test materials. Contact Dermatitis. 1998;39:68–70.
69. Cyran C, Maibach H. Alternate vehicles for diagnostic patch testing: an update. G Ital Dermatol Venereol. 2008;143(2):91–4.
70. Fischer T, Maibach HI. The thin layer rapid use epicutaneous test (TRUE-test), a new patch test method with high accuracy. Br J Dermatol. 1984;112:63–8.
71. Kreilgard B, Hansen J. Aspects of pharmaceutical and chemical standardization of patch test materials. J Am Acad Dermatol. 1989;21:836–8.
72. Kim HO, Wester RC, McMaster JA, Bucks DA, Maibach HI. Skin absorption from patch test systems. Contact Dermatitis. 1987;17:178–80.
73. Fischer T, Maibach HI. Amount of nickel applied with a standard patch test. Contact Dermatitis. 1984;11:285–7.
74. Bruze M, Isaksson M, Gruvberger B, Frick-Engfeldt M. Recommendation of appropriate amounts of petrolatum preparation to be applied at patch testing. Contact Dermatitis. 2007;56:281–5.
75. Antoine JL, Lachapelle JM. Variations in the quantities of petrolatum applied in patch testing. Derm Beruf Umwelt. 1988;36:191–4.
76. Bruze M, Frick-Engfeldt M, Gruvberger B, Isaksson M. Variation in the amount of petrolatum preparation applied at patch testing. Contact Dermatitis. 2007;56:38–42.
77. Shaw DW, Zhai H, Maibach HI, Niklasson B. Dosage considerations in patch testing with liquid allergens. Contact Dermatitis. 2002;47:86–90.
78. Kimber I, Gerberick GF, Basketter DA. Thresholds in contact sensitization: theoretical and practical considerations. Food Chem Toxicol. 1999;37:553–60.
79. Allenby CF, Basketter DA. Minimum eliciting patch test concentrations of cobalt. Contact Dermatitis. 1989;20:185–90.
80. Johansen Duus J, Andersen KE, Rastogi SC, Menné T. Threshold responses in cinnamic aldehyde sensitive subjects: results and methodological aspects. Contact Dermatitis. 1996;34:165–71.
81. Johansen Duus J, Andersen KE, Menné T. Quantitative aspects of isoeugenol contact allergy assessed by use and patch tests. Contact Dermatitis. 1996;34:414–8.
82. Maibach HI. Diagnostic patch test concentration for Kathon CG. Contact Dermatitis. 1985;13:242–5.
83. Zaghi D, Maibach HI. Quantitative relationships between patch test reactivity and use test reactivity: an overview. Cutan Ocul Toxicol. 2008;27(3):241–8.
84. Pontén A, Aalto-Korte K, Agner T, Andersen KE, Giménez-Arnau AM, Gonçalo M, et al. Patch testing with 2.0 % (0.60 mg/cm 2) formaldehyde instead of 1.0 % (0.30 mg/cm 2) detects significantly more contact allergy. Contact Dermatitis. 2013;68(1):50–3.
85. Nethercott J. Practical problems in the use of patch test in the evaluation of patients with contact dermatitis. Curr Probl Dermatol. 1990;4:101–23.
86. Menné T, Christophersen J, Maibach HI. Epidemiology of allergic contact sensitization. Monogr Allergy. 1987;21:132–61.
87. Christophersen J, Menné T, Tanghøj P, Andersen KE, Brandrup F, Kaaber K, et al. Clinical patch test data evaluated by multivariate analysis. Danish Contact Dermatitis Group. Contact Dermatitis. 1989;21(5):291–9.
88. Wilkinson DS, Fregert S, Magnusson B, Bandmann HJ, Calnan CD, Cronin E, et al. Terminology of contact dermatitis. Acta Derm Venereol. 1970;50(4):287–92.
89. Menné T, White I. Standardization in contact dermatitis. Contact Dermatitis. 2008;58:321.
90. Ivens U, Serup J, O'Gosh K. Allergy patch test reading from photographic images: disagreement on ICDRG grading but agreement on simplified tripartite reading. Skin Res Technol. 2007;13:110–3.
91. Bruze M, Isaksson M, Edman B, Björkner B, Fregert S, Möller H. A study on expert reading of patch test reactions: inter-individual accordance. Contact Dermatitis. 1995;32(6):331–7.

92. Ale SI, Maibach HI. 24-Hour versus 48-hour occlusion in patch testing. Exog Dermatol. 2003;2:270–6.
93. Mathias CGT, Maibach HI. When to read a patch test? Int J Dermatol. 1979;18:127–8.
94. Mitchell JC. Day 7 (D7) patch test reading—valuable or not? Contact Dermatitis. 1978;4:139–41.
95. Macfarlane AW, Curley RK, Graham RM, Lewis-Jones MS, King CM. Delayed patch test reactions at days 7 and 9. Contact Dermatitis. 1989;20:127–32.
96. Davis MD, Bhate K, Rohlinger AL, Farmer SA, Richardson DM, Weaver AL. Delayed patch test reading after 5 days: the Mayo Clinic experience. J Am Acad Dermatol. 2008;59: 225–33.
97. Fisher A, Dorman RL. The clinical significance of weak positive patch test reactions to certain allergens. Cutis. 1973;11:450–3. 151.
98. Vestergaard L, Clemmensen OJ, Sorensen FB, Andersen KE. Histological distinction between early allergic and irritant patch test reactions: follicular spongiosis may be characteristic of early allergic contact dermatitis. Contact Dermatitis. 1999;41:207–10.
99. Berardesca E, Maibach HI. Bioengineering and the patch test. Contact Dermatitis. 1988;18:3–9.
100. Serup J, Staberg B. Ultrasound for assessment of allergic and irritant patch test reactions. Contact Dermatitis. 1987;17:80–4.
101. Staberg B, Serup J. Allergic and irritant skin reactions evaluated by laser Doppler flowmetry. Contact Dermatitis. 1988;18:40–5.
102. Wahlberg JE, Wahlberg ENG. Quantification of skin blood flow at patch test sites. Contact Dermatitis. 1987;17:229–33.
103. Marzulli FN, Maibach HI. The use of graded concentrations in studying skin sensitizers: experimental contact sensitization in man. Food Cosmet Toxicol. 1974;12:219–27.
104. Koehler A, Maibach HI. Skin hyporeactivity in relation to patch testing. Contact Dermatitis. 2000;42:1–4.
105. Gollhausen R, Przybilla B, Ring J. Reproducibility of patch tests. J Am Acad Dermatol. 1989;21:1196–202.
106. Brasch J, Henseler T, Aberer W, Bäuerle G, Frosch PJ, Fuchs T, et al. Reproducibility of patch tests. A multicenter study of synchronous left-versus right-sided patch tests by the German Contact Dermatitis Research Group. J Am Acad Dermatol. 1994;31:584–91.
107. Lindelöf B. A left versus right side comparison study of Finn Chamber patch test in 200 consecutive patients. Contact Dermatitis. 1990;22:288–9.
108. Bousema MT, Geursen AM, van Joost TH. High reproducibility of patch tests [letter]. J Am Acad Dermatol. 1991;24:322.
109. Bourke JF, Batta K, Prais L, Abdullah A, Foulds IS. The reproducibility of patch tests. Br J Dermatol. 1999;140:102–5.
110. Lachapelle J-M. A left versus right side comparative study of Epiquick patch test results in 100 consecutive patients. Contact Dermatitis. 1989;20:51–5.
111. Ale SI, Maibach HI. Reproducibility of patch test reactions. A right versus left study using True Test. Contact Dermatitis. 2004;50:304–12.
112. Lachapelle JM. A proposed relevance scoring system for positive allergic patch test reactions: practical implications and limitations. Contact Dermatitis. 1997;36:39–43.
113. Ale SI, Maibach HI. Clinical relevance in allergic contact dermatitis. An algorithmic approach. Dermatol Beruf Umw. 1995;43:119–21.

"Doctor, Why Are My Patch Tests Negative?"

5

Denis Sasseville

> *Adopting the right attitude can convert a negative stress into a positive one.*
>
> *Hans Selye*

Not every patient referred for patch testing will end up with positive reactions. In his analysis of the cost-effectiveness of patch testing, Rietschel states that only about 53 % of patients suspected to have contact dermatitis will have one or more positive patch tests [1]. He also believes that a range of positive reactions between 30 and 65 % means appropriate utilization of patch testing. A yield below 30 % represents inadequate selection of patients and overuse of patch testing facilities. On the other hand, if the positivity rate is above 65 %, the patch testing physician is probably too selective and will likely not test many patients who would benefit from the procedure [1].

It is therefore quite normal that approximately half of patients undergoing patch testing will have no reaction. However, in a patient with true allergic contact dermatitis, patch testing may at times be falsely negative. This chapter will explore the causes of negative patch tests and give advice in order to maximize the yield of the procedure while avoiding false-negative reactions. The approach to the patient with negative tests will also be discussed.

D. Sasseville, MD, FRCPC
Division of Dermatology, Department of Medicine,
McGill University Health Centre, Royal Victoria Hospital,
Room A4.17, 687 Pine Avenue West,
Montréal, QC H3A 1A1, Canada
e-mail: denis.sasseville@mcgill.ca

J.-M. Lachapelle et al. (eds.), *Patch Testing Tips*,
DOI 10.1007/978-3-642-45395-3_5, © Springer-Verlag Berlin Heidelberg 2014

5.1   True-Negative Reactions

5.1.1   Not Contact Dermatitis

Patients with endogenous eczema such as atopic dermatitis, neurodermatitis, pompholyx, or stasis dermatitis are often referred for patch testing. These patients often have used numerous topical preparations to which they may have become sensitized. The procedure is indicated when the condition is long-standing, poorly responding to treatment, or localized to specific areas such as the eyelids, hands and feet, perianal area, or around leg ulcers, situations suggesting superimposed contact allergy. At times, patients with noneczematous conditions may need to be tested. These may include subjective ailments such as orodynia or vulvodynia or visible lesions of oral or cutaneous lichenoid reactions, eczematized psoriasis, and id reactions secondary to tinea pedis, etc. Under these circumstances, the physician is more or less expecting a negative reaction, and such a result does not come as a surprise.

5.1.2   Irritant Contact Dermatitis

Examples of contact dermatitis caused by exposure to strong or mild irritants include chemical burns, dermatitis caused by repeated hand washing, frictional dermatitis, and asteatotic eczema. These cases represent between 70 and 80 % of all cases of contact dermatitis [2]. Often, the diagnosis can be suspected based on the subacute to chronic morphology of the lesions, the predominance of burning pain over pruritus, and the history of exposure to known irritants. Some notorious irritants (formaldehyde, glutaral, metal salts, many biocides, etc.) are also potential allergens, and patch tests may be necessary to establish the distinction between irritant and allergic contact dermatitis or to prove the presence of both conditions. The importance of patch testing becomes paramount when dealing with occupational or medicolegal cases. Here again, negative patch testing is the expected result.

5.2   False-Negative Reactions

The causes of falsely negative patch tests are numerous and should always be kept in mind to avoid labeling patients as nonallergic when, in fact, they have an undiagnosed and easily curable condition. The consequences of such a misdiagnosis are more profound and far-reaching than those of a false-positive reaction, because patients will be prone to multiple recurrences of their dermatitis when they are reexposed to offending allergens.

5.2.1   Missed Allergen

This situation is the most common cause of negative patch tests in the presence of contact allergy. It occurs when a patient has not been tested to his allergen and could therefore be called a "false false-negative reaction." Contact dermatitis should be considered allergic until proven otherwise by comprehensive patch testing. Baseline series should be relied on as screening tools only. Larkin and Rietschel have shown that the European standard series will detect at best about 65 % of cases of allergic contact dermatitis [3]. More recently, Patel and Belsito, in a retrospective study of 2,088 patch-tested patients, found that only 27.6 % would have been fully evaluated by the two-panel TRUE Test and that 13.1 % would have been totally missed when tested to the more comprehensive North American Contact Dermatitis Group (NACDG) standard series of 65 allergens [4]. These screening tools need to be supplemented by additional series and personal products that reflect patients' exposures. When dealing with occupational contact dermatitis, it is imperative to review the composition of every product that may be deposited on the skin by direct or airborne exposure and to test patients with adequately prepared samples of workplace products [5].

5.2.2 Technical Failure

Patch testing is the gold standard, time-honored technique to diagnose contact allergy. It is well known, however, that its results are not always reproducible [6, 7]. Even when properly performed, the technique remains a rather crude bioassay that does not exactly mimic real-life conditions: a 48-h application on intact skin, even under occlusion, is not equivalent to daily applications over large areas or on damaged integument. When allergy is strongly suspected, additional procedures such as repeat open application tests (ROATs), use tests, semi-open tests, scratch patch tests, or patch tests preceded by tape stripping may reveal sensitizers when regular patch testing is negative [8]. In addition, a number of technical errors may supervene and result in falsely negative tests [9, 10].

5.2.2.1 Insufficient Occlusion
The patch test strips may fall off or become loose if they have not been properly secured to the back. If they have not been applied with the patient sitting or standing in a neutral position, they may wrinkle or rip off when the patient straightens or bends. Extra tape may be required to ensure proper occlusion, especially in hot and humid weather conditions.

5.2.2.2 Insufficient Duration of Application
It is generally recommended to occlude the patches for 48 h in order to promote adequate penetration of the allergen. For years, numerous investigators have tried to compare the results of patch testing using different occlusion times [11–15]. Most of these parallel studies have shown no significant differences between occlusion times of 24 versus 48 h, even though some have not demonstrated perfectly concordant results [11, 12]. Positive reactions occurring only after 24-h occlusion periods were seen as often as those appearing only after 48 h. Later studies yielded concordant results in 86 and 93.3 % of the cases, respectively [13, 14]. They were, however, conducted on a relatively small number of patients, 15 in the Goh et al. study and 236 in the Macháčková and Seda study. A much larger multicenter, unpaired study involving 15,553 patients showed a statistically significant difference in the

reaction index when patches were applied for 24 or 48 h. The shorter application time gave better results and was associated with a lesser number of irritant reactions [15]. Commenting on previously published studies, Manuskiatti and Maibach state that no definite conclusion could be drawn and that it appears premature to recommend a 24-h application time as long as additional studies are not carried out in an ideal experimental design [16].

5.2.2.3 Insufficient Amount of Allergen

The ideal amount of a standardized, petrolatum-based allergen should be 20 mg per patch, corresponding to a strip, extruded from the syringe, that covers the diameter of an 8-mm Finn Chamber[hyo0] [17]. False-negative reactions may also occur when the patch test technician, distracted by ambient conversations, forgets to fill a test chamber or fails to warn the attending physician that an allergen has run out. Maintenance of a constant supply of allergens and provision of a quiet environment for the preparation of the patches will reduce or eliminate these sources of errors.

5.2.2.4 Insufficient Concentration of Allergen

This situation is likely to arise when testing nonstandard allergens such as workplace chemicals or patients' personal products and topical medicaments. Diluting a product in order to avoid triggering an irritant reaction may render the final concentration of the offending allergen too low to elicit a positive reaction. Cosmetics that cause allergic contact dermatitis under real-life, daily usage may fail to react when patch tested for 48 h. Testing with a patient's own antibiotic preparation may be falsely negative because the concentration required to bring out a positive patch test reaction on intact skin is often 20–40 times that found in the finished product. This is why neomycin, framycetin, gentamicin, and bacitracin are tested at concentrations of 20 % in petrolatum. Rycroft correctly points out that "the first insurance against false-negative reactions is therefore the use of standardized patch test materials of reliable reactivity" [18]. Products brought by patients need to be prepared in nonirritant concentrations and mixed in the appropriate vehicle, according to existing literature [19]. When information is not available, multiple dilutions and vehicles must be used, as well as a number of controls.

5.2.2.5 Inactive Allergen

To induce allergic contact dermatitis, some chemicals must be oxidized. This is the case for D-limonene, tea tree oil, turpentine, linalool, etc. The substance used for patch testing therefore needs to be in the same oxidized state to reveal the allergic sensitization [20–22]. Many commercially available allergens such as metal salts are quite stable, but others degrade very easily and can disappear within days or even hours if kept at room temperature or applied in advance to test chambers. Such is the case with numerous isocyanates and acrylates that should be ideally stored in the freezer and thawed just prior to application [23, 24]. Additional examples of substances that may not be stable forever include corticosteroids, formaldehyde, sodium hypochlorite, and paraphenylenediamine. Every allergen should be refrigerated if not frozen and stored in the dark. Expiration dates should be respected, and allergens replaced in a timely manner in order to avoid falsely negative tests due to inexistent allergens.

5.2.2.6 Inadequate Vehicle

Penetration of the allergen in the epidermis may be impaired if the allergen is not released from the vehicle in which it is mixed. Negative patch tests to hydrocortisone-17-butyrate and other corticosteroids may be the result of testing in petrolatum instead of ethanol [25]. Acyclovir and minoxidil need to be tested in propylene glycol to elicit positive reactions [26, 27].

5.2.2.7 Compound Allergy

This term refers to the situation where a patient shows a positive patch test reaction to a product while testing of its individual ingredients remains negative [28, 29]. True compound allergy has rarely been documented. It may result from the interaction, inside the product, of separate ingredients to produce a new allergen or from metabolic transformation of one or more ingredients by cutaneous enzymes. Pseudocompound allergy is probably more common and may be due to irritancy of the finished product or to the selection of inadequate concentrations when testing the individual ingredients.

5.2.3 Patient-Related Failure

As an active participant in the testing procedure, the patient must understand and follow the given instructions. He or she must avoid sweating, showering, and exercising lest the patch test strips come loose, making the whole process a useless exercise. It is therefore important to meet patients beforehand for a verbal explanation of the patch test technique and to provide them with a written handout to refresh their memory, especially if there is a certain amount of delay between the initial visit and actual testing.

The damping effect of immunosuppression on patch testing reactivity should not be underestimated. It is at times necessary to test mildly or profoundly immunosuppressed patients. There is a general feeling among experts in contact dermatitis that if an immunosuppressed patient presents with active lesions of allergic contact dermatitis, he is still capable of mounting an immune reaction and patch tests should be positive. Patches should be applied on intact skin, and the site of application should not have been previously treated with topical corticosteroids, as these agents are known to dampen or suppress reactions [30, 31]. Members of the NACDG feel that topical application of corticosteroids should be avoided over the test site at least 3–7 days prior to patch testing [32].

The effect of systemic corticosteroid on patch testing reactions has also been evaluated [33–37]. O'Quinn tested 20 patients with known contact allergies and found that the administration of 40 mg of prednisone abolished reactions in 6 of them and diminished the intensity of reactions in 6 other individuals [33]. Suppressed reactions again became positive when the dose of prednisone was lowered to 20 mg. It should be noted that the initial reactions, off prednisone, were strongly positive. It is therefore possible that weak reactions could still be suppressed by the lower dose of prednisone. Feuerman and Levy found that a daily dose of 40 mg suppressed reactions in 3 of 12 patients, while 20 mg abolished reactivity in only 1 of

16 subjects [34]. After administration of an oral dose of 40 mg of prednisone, Condie and Adams were unable to suppress patch test reactions to *Rhus* antigen [35]. Urushiol is a notoriously potent allergen, however, and from this study no conclusion can be drawn on the effect of such a dose of prednisone on weak reactions. A recent multicenter study evaluated the outcome of nickel-allergic patients tested twice with nickel sulfate while on placebo and while receiving a daily dose of prednisone 20 mg [37]. There was a significant reduction in the total number of positive reactions from 171 on placebo to 63 on prednisone. In those who still reacted, there was a shift from strong to weak or doubtful reactions. Members of the NACDG believe that patients submitted to patch testing should not be taking a daily dose of more than 10 mg of prednisone [32].

The effect of other systemic immunosuppressants on patch test reactivity is less well known. Wee et al. patch tested 38 patients who were taking azathioprine, methotrexate, cyclosporine, tacrolimus, mycophenolate mofetil, and the TNF-α inhibitors etanercept, infliximab, and adalimumab. Seventeen patients displayed reactions varying from + to +++. The authors conclude that, when indicated, patch testing should not be postponed in patients taking immunosuppressive drugs. Given that the allergic status of their patients prior to the introduction of immunosuppressants was unknown, they also state that "this study could not, however, shed light on what degree some allergic reactions may have been suppressed by particular immunomodulating drugs" [38]. Of the 11 patients tested while on immunosuppressants by Rosmarin et al., 10 had positive reactions graded + to +++ [39]. Only one patient, on mycophenolate mofetil, was retested after the drug was discontinued and showed positive reactions to formaldehyde, formaldehyde releasers, and MCI/MI that were not detected during the initial testing session. More recently, it was shown that ustekinumab, an inhibitor of interleukins 12 and 23, was ineffective in the treatment of allergic contact dermatitis and had no effect on patch testing [40, 41]. From the preceding studies, one can conclude that false-negative reactions can occur when testing patients taking immunosuppressants but that the risk may be less with biological immunomodulators.

Ultraviolet light irradiation is known to locally decrease the number of Langerhans cells and also induce a state of systemic immunosuppression susceptible to suppress weak patch test reactions [42]. It is recommended to avoid exposure to natural or artificial sources of ultraviolet light between 2 and 4 weeks prior to patch testing [32, 43]. Patients taking pentoxifylline, a methylxanthine derivative that has inhibitory activity against TNF-α, have been shown to experience a decrease in patch test response that could result in false-negative testing [44, 45]. A similar state of hyporeactivity has been alluded to with cimetidine, H1-antihistamines, diltiazem, and pentamidine [46].

5.2.4 Physician-Related Failure

Any health professional undertaking patch testing should have an in-depth knowledge of the pathophysiology of allergic contact dermatitis and of the methodology of patch testing, thereby minimizing or avoiding potential sources of false-negative reactions as described below.

5.2.4.1 Too Early Testing

The experienced patch tester knows that he needs to "treat first, test later" in order to avoid false-positive reaction or the occurrence of the "angry back syndrome." It is a less well-known fact that testing in the presence of active dermatitis can also lead to false-negative reactions [47, 48]. It appears that cutaneous inflammation, whether induced by irritant or allergic mechanisms, may induce changes in the composition of the thickness and barrier function of the epidermis, leading to hyporeactivity that may last up to 9 weeks [48].

5.2.4.2 Too Late Testing

With time, the number of memory or primed effector T cells may decrease, especially if the allergen responsible for the initial sensitization is rarely encountered. Testing months or years after an episode of allergic contact dermatitis may fail to elicit a positive reaction. The procedure, however, can awaken a dormant immune system, and retesting a few weeks later may then bring forth a positive reaction.

5.2.4.3 Failure to Perform Early Readings

When the patient's history suggests contact urticaria, open or occluded patch tests need to be closely watched, every 10–20 min for up to 2–3 h, lest an immediate reaction be missed if the tests are read in the usual fashion after 48 and 96 h.

5.2.4.4 Failure to Perform Late Readings

A single reading at 48 h, when patches are removed, will fail to reveal 25–30 % of positive reactions. Readings at 96 h should always be performed. Some allergens, such as corticosteroids and neomycin, are notorious late reactors that may become positive only after 5–7 days.

5.2.4.5 Failure to Perform Specific Procedures

The allergens responsible for photocontact dermatitis need to be activated by ultraviolet light to induce sensitization. Proceeding with patch testing instead of photopatch testing in such cases will obviously translate in false-negative results. Similarly, failure to perform prick testing in cases of protein contact dermatitis or a stepwise combination of patch, prick, and intradermal testing in cases of adverse drug eruptions will also lead to falsely negative tests.

5.3 Approach to the Patch Test-Negative Patient

All patients are anxious to find the cause of their dermatitis. The best case scenario is when patch testing uncovers one or more allergens that are easy to avoid and are the cause of the patient's condition. In this case, avoidance is synonymous with cure, and everyone is happy, including the physician, who envisions a publication if he has discovered a new allergen. Patients who are told that their patch tests are negative will display a wide range of emotions [49]. Some will be beaming with joy and relief, especially those who feared that a positive test would make them lose their job or prevent them from receiving a metallic implant. For the majority, however, the news of negative testing is a source of disappointment and frustration, often manifested by incredulity, sadness, and sometimes tears or anger, always accompanied by multiple questions, especially from those who have scribbled on their referral note "you are my last hope." They will often ask if more tests can be done, what is the cause of their condition if there is no external cause, how can it be cured, etc. Often, they see themselves in a dead end, with an incurable, lifelong disease.

Prevention should begin early, as soon as patch testing is considered. It should be emphasized to the patient that there are many causes of dermatitis and that, sometimes, different conditions may overlap. A careful preliminary history and physical examination are mandatory and will help establish a diagnosis of endogenous eczema or other personal dermatosis. When patch testing appears justified, it is important to explain not only the technique but also the purpose of the test. Patients should be told that patch tests will only disclose contact allergies but not irritant contact dermatitis or food and inhalant allergies. When looking for allergic contact dermatitis superimposed on endogenous eczema, it is imperative to warn patients that finding and eliminating contact allergens may help but not cure their condition. They will therefore come to the patch testing session with more realistic expectations and hopefully will not be floored by negative results.

Conclusion

Any patient with negative patch testing should be reassessed. The history should be reviewed, in search of a missed allergen from the workplace, household, or hobbies. Potential causes of false-negative reactions should not be overlooked and additional procedures such as repeat patch testing, photopatch and prick testing, ROATs, skin biopsy and cultures, etc., undertaken as needed. When the investigation is complete and the final diagnosis is one of endogenous eczema, it will be necessary to provide support, hope, and guidance. Patients need to be told that, even though there is no cure for their disease, it can be treated and often well controlled with adequate treatment. I often tell patients who have been suffering over many years from recurrent bouts of eczema that they did not have this condition during all of their past life and that it is very likely that they will experience long-lasting periods of remission. I also tell them that neither they nor I can predict the future and that we need to tackle the problem one day at a time. At that point, many patients will feel reassured that patch testing, even if it ended up being negative, was not done in vain.

Practical Tips
- Make sure to look for and test every possible allergen that your patient is exposed to.
- Use comprehensive series of standardized allergens.
- Prepare nonstandardized allergens in appropriate concentrations and vehicles.
- Perform early and late readings, photopatch tests, prick tests, and repeat open application tests and use tests as the situation requires.
- Do not hesitate to repeat procedures if your working diagnosis remains allergic contact dermatitis.

References

1. Rietschel RL. Is patch testing cost-effective? J Am Acad Dermatol. 1989;21:885–7.
2. Nosbaum A, Vocanson M, Rozières A, Hennino A, Nicolas JF. Allergic and irritant contact dermatitis. Eur J Dermatol. 2009;19(4):1–8.
3. Larkin A, Rietschel RL. The utility of patch testing using larger screening series of allergens. Am J Contact Dermat. 1998;9:142–5.
4. Patel D, Belsito DV. The detection of clinically relevant contact allergens with a standard screening tray of 28 allergens. Contact Dermatitis. 2012;66:154–8.
5. Rycroft RJG. Problems in occupational allergy. Semin Dermatol. 1982;1:43–7.
6. Gollhausen R, Przybilla B, Ring J. Reproducibility of patch tests. J Am Acad Dermatol. 1989;21:1196–202.
7. Brasch J, Henseler T, Aberer W, Baüerle G, Frosch PJ, Fuchs T, et al. Reproducibility of patch tests. A multicenter study of synchronous left versus right-sided patch tests by the German Contact Dermatitis Research Group. J Am Acad Dermatol. 1994;31:584–91.
8. Lachapelle JM, Maibach HI. Additional testing procedures and spot tests. In: Lachapelle JM, Maibach HI, editors. Patch testing and prick testing. 3rd ed. Berlin/Heidelberg: Springer; 2012. p. 113–28.
9. Rietschel RL, Fowler Jr JF. Fisher's contact dermatitis. 6th ed. Hamilton: B.C. Decker Inc; 2008. p. 15.
10. Lindberg M, Matura M. Patch testing. In: Johansen JD, Frosch PJ, Lepoittevin JP, editors. Contact dermatitis. 5th ed. Berlin/Heidelberg: Springer; 2011. p. 439–64.
11. Skog E, Forsbeck M. Comparison between 24- and 48-h exposure time in patch testing. Contact Dermatitis. 1978;4:362–4.
12. Kalimo K, Lammintausta K. 24- and 48-h allergen exposure in patch testing. Comparative study with 11 common contact allergens and NiCl2. Contact Dermatitis. 1984;10:25–9.
13. Goh CL, Wong WK, Ng SK. Comparison between 1-day and 2-day occlusion times in patch testing. Contact Dermatitis. 1994;31:48–50.
14. Macháčková J, Seda O. Reproducibility of patch tests. J Am Acad Dermatol. 1991;25:732–3.
15. Brasch J, Geier J, Henseler T. Evaluation of patch test results by use of the reaction index. An analysis of data recorded by the Information Network of Departments of Dermatology (IVDK). Contact Dermatitis. 1995;33:375–80.
16. Manuskiatti W, Maibach HI. 1- versus 2- and 3-day diagnostic patch testing. Contact Dermatitis. 1996;35:197–200.
17. Bruze M, Isaksson M, Gruvberger B, Frick-Engfeldt M. Recommendations of appropriate amounts of petrolatum preparations to be applied at patch testing. Contact Dermatitis. 2007; 56:281–5.
18. Rycroft RJG. False reactions to nonstandard patch tests. Semin Dermatol. 1986;5:225–30.
19. De Groot A. Patch testing. Test concentrations and vehicles for 4350 chemicals. 3rd ed. Amsterdam: AC Degroot Publishing; 2008.
20. Matura M, Sköld M, Börje A, Andersen KE, Bruze M, Frosch P, et al. Selected oxidized fragrance terpenes are common contact allergens. Contact Dermatitis. 2005;52:320–8.
21. Hausen BM. Evaluation of the main contact allergens in oxidized tea tree oil. Dermatitis. 2004;15:213–4.
22. Sköld M, Börje A, Harambasic E, Karlberg AT. Contact allergens formed on air exposure of linalool. Identification and quantification of primary and secondary oxidation products and the effect on skin sensitization. Chem Res Toxicol. 2004;17:1697–705.
23. Frick M, Zimerson E, Karlsson D, Marand A, Skarping G, Isaksson M, et al. Poor correlation between stated an found concentrations of diphenyl methane-4,4'-diisocyanate (4,4"-MDI) in petrolatum patch test preparations. Contact Dermatitis. 2004;51:73–8.
24. Mose KF, Andersen KE, Christensen LP. Stability of selected volatile contact allergens in different patch test chambers under different storage conditions. Contact Dermatitis. 2012;66: 172–9.
25. Wilkinson SM, Beck MH. Corticosteroid contact hypersensitivity: what vehicle and concentration? Contact Dermatitis. 1996;34:305–8.

26. Serpentier-Daude A, Collet E, Didier AF, Touraud JP, Sgro C, Lambert D. Dermites de contact aux antiherpétiques locaux. Ann Dermatol Venereol. 2000;127:191–3.
27. Whitmore SE. The importance of proper vehicle selection in the detection of minoxidil sensitivity. Arch Dermatol. 1992;128:653–6.
28. Kellet JK, King CM, Beck MH. Compound allergy to medicaments. Contact Dermatitis. 1986;14:45–8.
29. Le Coz CJ, Sasseville D. Interprétation et pertinence des patch tests: faux positifs et faux négatifs, allergies composées, allergies croisées. Ann Dermatol Venereol. 2009;136:610–6.
30. Sukanto H, Nater JP, Bleumink E. Influence of topically applied corticosteroids on patch test reactions. Contact Dermatitis. 1981;7:180–5.
31. Clark R, Rietschel R. The effect of triamcinolone acetonide ointment 0.1% on positive patch tests. Arch Dermatol. 1982;118:163–5.
32. Fowler Jr JF, Maibach HI, Taylor JS, DeKoven JG, Sasseville D, Warshaw EM, et al. Effects of immunomodulatory agents on patch testing: expert opinion 2012. Dermatitis. 2012;23:301–3.
33. O'Quinn SE, Isbell KH. Influence of oral prednisone on eczematous patch test reactions. Arch Dermatol. 1969;99:380–9.
34. Feuerman E, Levy A. A study of the effect of prednisone and an antihistamine on patch test reactions. Br J Dermatol. 1972;86:68–71.
35. Condie MW, Adams RM. Influence of oral prednisone on patch test reactions to Rhus antigen. Arch Dermatol. 1973;107:540–3.
36. Olupona T, Scheinman P. Successful patch testing despite concomitant low-dose prednisone use. Dermatitis. 2008;19:117–8.
37. Anveden I, Lindberg M, Andersen KE, Bruze M, Isaksson M, Liden C, et al. Oral prednisone suppresses allergic but not irritant patch test reactions in individuals hypersensitive to nickel. Contact Dermatitis. 2004;50:298–303.
38. Wee JS, White JML, McFadden JP, White IR. Patch testing in patients treated with systemic immunosuppression and cytokine inhibitors. Contact Dermatitis. 2010;62:165–9.
39. Rosmarin D, Gottlieb AB, Asarch A, Scheinman PL. Patch-testing while on systemic immunosuppressant's. Dermatitis. 2009;20:265–70.
40. Bangsgaard N, Zachariae C, Menné T, Skov L. Lack of effect of ustekinumab in treatment of allergic contact dermatitis. Contact Dermatitis. 2011;65:227–30.
41. Nosbaum A, Rozières A, Balme B, Goujon C, Nicolas JF, Bérard F. Blocking T helper 1/T helper 17 pathways has no effect on patch testing. Contact Dermatitis. 2013;68:58–9.
42. Cruz PD. Effects of UV light on the immune system: answer to five basic questions. Am J Contact Dermat. 1996;7:47–52.
43. Lachapelle JM, Maibach HI. Patch testing methodology. In: Lachapelle JM, Maibach HI, editors. Patch testing and prick testing. 3rd ed. Berlin/Heidelberg: Springer; 2012. p. 35–77.
44. Schwarz T, Schwarz A, Krone C, Luger TA. Pentoxifylline suppresses allergic patch test reactions in humans. Arch Dermatol. 1993;129:513–4.
45. Balato N, Patruno C, Lembo G, Cuccurullo FM, Ayala F. Effect of pentoxifylline on patch test response. Contact Dermatitis. 1996;34:153.
46. Collet E, Didier AF. Ce qu'il ne faut jamais faire en dermato-allergologie. In: Le Coz CJ, Jelen G, Lepoittevin JP, editors. Progrès en dermato-allergologie- Strasbourg 2003. Paris: John Libbey Eurotext; 2003. p. 153–9.
47. Lammintausta K, Maibach HI. Human cutaneous irritation: induced hyporeactivity. Contact Dermatitis. 1987;17:193–8.
48. Koehler AM, Maibach HI. Skin hyporeactivity in relation to patch testing. Contact Dermatitis. 2000;42:1–4.
49. Beck MH. The patient with negative patch tests – what now? In: Guin JD, editor. Practical contact dermatitis. New York: McGraw-Hill Inc; 1995. p. 659–72.

How to Select Extra Allergens and Problematic Allergens

6

Klaus Ejner Andersen

6.1 Introduction

The diagnosis of allergic contact dermatitis is based on a positive diagnostic patch test combined with the patient's history and the clinical pattern of the dermatitis. Contact allergy plays a role in about 35–40 % of patients with hand eczema [1]. Contact dermatitis is often a chronic and recurrent disease of multifactorial origin involving endogenous and exogenous factors. The choice of patch test allergens to be tested in a patient with suspected allergic contact dermatitis is crucial – for both occupationally and nonoccupationally related contact dermatitis. The correct diagnosis of allergic contact dermatitis may be missed if the allergen in question is not tested. The failure of diagnosing a contact allergy may have legal implications for occupationally related contact dermatitis and may affect the advice to the patient, the treatment, and prognosis of the eczema. The fact that allergic contact dermatitis is often a complicating factor aggravating other eczematous diseases adds to the uncertainty.

An experienced dermatologist may guess correctly the clinically important contact allergy in some patients. The guess may sometimes be correct for common allergens as nickel and is much more often incorrect for less common allergens (<10 %) [1–3].

The use of a baseline patch test series comprising the most common allergens in all patients with suspected allergic contact dermatitis is widely accepted. The baseline series may vary from clinic to clinic depending on what the population is exposed to, which may differ between geographic regions, the industrial development, and common occurrence of various professions and consumer goods and habits.

K.E. Andersen, MD, DMSc
Department of Dermatology and Allergy Centre,
Odense University Hospital, University of Southern Denmark,
Sdr. Boulevard 29, Odense 5000, Denmark
e-mail: keandersen@health.sdu.dk

J.-M. Lachapelle et al. (eds.), *Patch Testing Tips*,
DOI 10.1007/978-3-642-45395-3_6, © Springer-Verlag Berlin Heidelberg 2014

However, supplementary tests with working materials, properly diluted, and extra allergens selected on the basis of patient history and known exposures are often required to assure the correct diagnosis. It is mandatory to carefully consider the choice of patch test concentration and vehicle when testing with materials that are not standardized [4].

A survey from four university clinics showed that 5–23 % of the patients in different clinics had contact allergies to compounds outside the former European standard series only [5]. If contact allergies are diagnosed early and early intervention is carried out, the prognosis may be better [6].

According to de Groot's monograph on patch testing [7], there are at least 4,350 known contact allergens. Every year, new chemicals are added to the list as possible contact allergens. Most clinics have available only a few allergens beyond the baseline series, and only dermatology departments with a special interest in contact dermatitis have a big selection of extra contact allergens available for routine use when indicated.

6.2   Supplementary Patch Test Allergens

These extra allergens may be purchased from the commercial patch test material suppliers (e.g., TROLAB Almirall Hermal GmbH, in Reinbek, Germany; Chemotechnique, in Vellinge, Sweden; and allergEAZE, SmartPractice, in Calgary, Canada), or the raw material may be acquired from different sources and made up in petrolatum in the proper patch test concentration at a pharmacy. The commercial patch test materials have a limited shelf life. Each syringe is labeled with a date of expiration, which varies between substances. Some have a short shelf life due to evaporation or chemical change (i.e., oxidation). Special allergens may be acquired from industry, chemical suppliers, manufacturers, and workplaces and need preparation in appropriate concentration and in an appropriate vehicle before they can be used for testing patients.

A crucial point is how to select extra allergens for the individual patient. Here, it is important to ask the patient to bring to the clinic safety data sheets of working materials, labels from working material containers with information about ingredients, and contact information for the manufacturer. Based on this information together with the patient history and interview, it is possible to trace exposure to chemicals and substances that are potential contact allergens.

An important exposure source is the topical remedies used by the patient at home and at work (i.e., all cosmetics, skin care products, gloves, and other protective gear). Testing with products used at home and at work often gives positive patch test reactions of importance for evaluation of the patient's dermatitis [8, 9].

6.3   The Allergen Bank

Rare allergens may also be acquired from an "allergen bank." This is an option in certain countries [10, 11] (www.allergenbanken.dk). The basic idea is to make available to dermatologists in private practice extra allergens, which he/she can order from the "bank" for specific testing of individual patients guided by the exposure history, obtained either through job description and the dermatologist's specific knowledge of allergen exposure or through evaluation of safety data sheets.

The allergen bank contains four separate parts:

1. A "bank," which is a refrigerator with about 400–500 numbered contact allergens obtained from commercial suppliers, product manufacturers, and pharmacies. The contact allergens are most often prepared in petrolatum and kept in polypropylene syringes in darkness at 4 °C. A few allergens are stored in bottles in appropriate vehicles and others in the freezer due to stability concerns.

2. A list of available contact allergens divided into appropriate series or lists of allergens from which the dermatologist can select extra allergens for an individual patient. The list is available to the dermatologist subscribing to the service in a booklet and on the password-protected website. The list is updated regularly and contains information about the source of the allergen, concentration and vehicle, CAS number when available, and other relevant information where appropriate (i.e., INCI names and synonym names).

3. A mailing system, so the contact allergens ordered from a dermatologist for a specific patient can be mailed shortly before scheduled patch testing in order to counteract stability problems present for volatile contact allergens as fragrance chemicals and acrylates [12, 13]. The allergens are shipped in plastic chambers with a lid (i.e., IQ chamber [Chemotechnique Diagnostics, Vellinge, Sweden]) or for volatile allergens in Van der Bend transport containers (Van der Bend BV, Brielle, the Netherlands), and it is highly recommended that the allergens are kept in a refrigerator until use.

4. A database, to register allergens, subscribing dermatologists, patch-tested patients, and the outcome of the tests. The subscribing dermatologist is obliged to supply relevant information for each patient tested with allergens ordered from the allergen bank. It encompasses personal identification number, age, sex, MOAHLFA index, and scheduled date for testing, and to send back to the allergen bank the result of the patch test procedure. Information about the relevance of the positive patch tests is also recorded when available. The program also contains a statistical package that makes it possible to extract patch test data in various ways according to research questions and quality control.

In Denmark, the allergen bank service supplying "rare" allergens to dermatologists, on a case-by-case basis, was established in 1992 [10, 11]. A similar service has been established in Australia [14], the Contact Allergen Bank Australia (http://www.occderm.asn.au/projects.html), and in the Netherlands (T. Rustemeyer, personal information, 2014). The extent of service and the organization of an allergen bank service depend on the organization of the local health care system in each country. Such a service carries advantages and also challenges, as pointed out in Table 6.1.

An allergen bank is a pragmatic tool for dermatologists interested in contact dermatitis, and the value of the "tool" is, of course, dependent on how it is used. The Danish Allergen Bank only accepts subscription from certified dermatologists in the country, and they are all to varying degrees trained in diagnostic patch testing. The interested and knowledgeable dermatologist can use the allergen bank service to provide optimal clinical evaluation and testing of contact dermatitis patients without

Table 6.1 The allergen bank: advantages and challenges

Advantages

Extra allergens are easily available for the dermatologist.

The patient may avoid referral to other clinic and thereby save time.

Improved diagnosis of contact allergy is possible.

More detailed testing and advice may improve prognosis of the dermatitis.

Occupational cases may be notified more carefully, and this may affect legal compensation.

Detection of "new" allergens in the environment is possible.

More experience with rare allergens, levels of test concentration, and level of irritancy.

The easy access to extra allergens makes diagnostic testing more rewarding for the dermatologist.

The service may be used as a quality control of patch test activity in the clinic.

The database included in the allergen bank is a research tool.

Challenges

The dermatologist should obtain an adequate patient history of exposure.

Relevant allergens should be ordered.

What is most efficient for optimal evaluation of the individual patient – testing with extra series of allergens based on exposure history or aimed testing with selected allergens based on exposure analysis?

Quality of allergens – regular renewal of patch test material is required.

Test results should be returned to the allergen bank for inclusion in the database.

Economy – annual subscription fee (600 €/year in Denmark) or payment per patch test.

having all relevant environmental contact allergens in stock in the clinic – and avoid referring these patients to another clinic. Other dermatologists may choose to omit testing beyond the baseline series and refer more "problematic" contact dermatitis patients to a tertiary center with the expertise and allergens available. The question arises: Who has the knowledge and experience required and who does not? That can be debated.

In Denmark about half of the dermatologists in private practice subscribe to the allergen bank.

Recently, two publications with data from the allergen bank service have been published. They report how dermatologists in private practice have identified patients with important and relevant contact allergies to thiourea compounds and to octylisothiazolinone [15, 16]. Some of these patients may have escaped diagnosis, information, and advice if the allergens had not been available through the bank service – or perhaps they would have been referred to a tertiary center, with the waiting time and overall expenses attached to the extra test procedures.

About 900–1,000 patients a year are tested with allergens ordered from the Danish Allergen Bank and a total of about 14,000–15,000 patch tests are mailed to the clinics, giving an estimated average of 14–15 allergens per patient. Most allergens are tested as part of a supplementary series, and about 15–20 % are ordered as single allergens for aimed testing of a specific patient.

The value of an allergen bank is, of course, questionable, and critics argue that the contact dermatitis patients are better off being referred to a tertiary center with more experience and "all" contact allergens available. The limitations for this opinion include, among other factors, waiting time, transport, more days off work, extra test procedures, and capacity at the tertiary center. The proponents for an allergen bank argue that contact dermatitis is an important subspecialty in dermatology, and dermatologists in practice should be able to perform diagnostic patch testing on a level beyond using a baseline series. In this case, an allergen bank is a pragmatic solution that gives the dermatologist access to extra allergens without keeping them in stock at the clinic. Many supplementary series are used rarely, and the allergens may soon reach the expiration date listed on the syringe. The allergen bank can deliver "fresh" allergens.

Further, the collection of patch test results in the database becomes an important source of information for clinical research. When the allergen bank service is in use in clinics around the country, it gives dermatologists an opportunity to discover new "small epidemics" of special contact allergies before they are perceived at the tertiary centers. It is the author's opinion that the allergen bank has a pedagogic influence, making the dermatologists in practice more interested in contact dermatitis – "it becomes professionally more rewarding to investigate contact dermatitis patients and to find the relevant allergies."

6.4   Information About Rare Allergens

Information about rare allergens can be obtained from the contact dermatitis textbooks. Further information can be obtained from valuable databases on the Internet such as PubMed and many others (see Table 6.2).

Further, An Goossens, Department of Dermatology, K.U. Leuven, Belgium, has developed the CDESKPRO website – http://www.cdeskpro.be – available to registered users with a large amount of information on allergens, topical pharmaceutical products, lists of cosmetic products not containing the specific allergens, literature references, and useful links. The website is available in English, French, and Dutch. Other national websites include the national contact dermatitis research groups and the European Contact Dermatitis Society (http://www.ESCD.org).

A simple, efficient approach sometimes is just to search the name of substance or the CAS number, when available, in Google or a similar search engine, and this will lead you to information about the chemicals in question. The international hazard data sheets on occupation give relevant information about the different hazards associated with special occupations. The International Clinical Safety Cards (ICSC) lead you to other databases where you can trace information. Composition of various protective clothing and gloves can also be found on the Internet (see Table 6.2).

It is important to realize that the intention and quality of information are very different from website to website.

These activities may be time-consuming, but they are very important for an optimal outcome of the evaluation, advice, and treatment of contact dermatitis cases.

The websites from the patch test material suppliers are also useful and updated on a regular basis.

Table 6.2 Selected websites for retrieving information about chemicals and products to which a dermatitis patient is exposed

PubMed	http://www.ncbi.nlm.nih.gov/pubmed
Safety datasheets may be retrieved from the Web, for example	
In German	http://www.wingis-online.de/wingisonline/
In English	http://www.ilo.org/dyn/icsc/showcard.home
Other comprehensive sources of information	
The European Commission database with information on cosmetic ingredients	http://ec.europa.eu/consumers/sectors/cosmetics/cosing/
NIOSH Pocket Guide to Chemical Hazards	http://www.cdc.gov/niosh/topics/chemical.html
Occupational Health Guidelines for Chemical Hazards	http://www.cdc.gov/niosh/topics/default.html
The German Institute of Occupational Safety and Health	http://www.dguv.de/ifa/en/index.jsp
List of allergens in protective gloves	http://www.bgbau.de/gisbau/service/allergene/allergeneliste-nach-hersteller-1
Environmental Health and Toxicology	http://sis.nlm.nih.gov/enviro.html
ChemIDplus contains information on chemistry and toxicity for 370,000 substances	http://chem.sis.nlm.nih.gov/chemidplus/chemidlite.jsp
Certain databases require subscription for access to the information	
ChemKnowledge	http://www.rightanswer.com/index.php/knowledge-solutions/chemknowledge-system/tomes-plus-system
CDESKPRO	http://www.cdeskpro.be/files/opties_e.htm

Searching can be time-consuming but is often worthwhile both for yourself and for your patients. With more training, you develop search strategies, which will ease your work.

6.5 "Difficult Allergens"

Chemical substances with a patch test concentration close to the irritant threshold concentration are difficult to test with because they may cause a high frequency of doubtful positive reactions, which may be a sign of irritancy or a weak positive allergic reaction. Emulsifiers, some biocides, and fragrance chemicals are examples of difficult allergens [17, 18]. When reading patch tests, it is often not possible to differentiate between a weak positive allergic reaction and an irritant reaction. In these cases, repeated patch tests, tests with a dilution series, late readings, and a careful exposure history may be helpful. These "difficult allergens" may also give rise to considerable variation between results from different clinics around the world. This variation may be partly explained by differences in scoring practices between dermatologists. In this context, it is important to acknowledge that diagnostic patch testing is just a tool for the dermatologist, with inherent pitfalls and variation due to several factors such as technical details, scoring of test results, and interindividual variation between patients and between dermatologists and that positive test results are not in themselves a result of current significant relevance without a thorough evaluation of the compound in question and the patient's history together with the clinical picture of the patient's dermatitis.

> **Practical Tips**
> - Contact allergy to substances beyond the baseline series is common.
> - Knowledge about exposure scenarios in various professions is important.
> - Safety data sheets for chemicals and list of ingredients in products are very helpful.
> - Guessing a patient's contact allergy is useless; testing is needed.
> - Patch test the patient with selected working material, topical remedies used, and protective gloves.
> - Rare allergens may be acquired from commercial patch test suppliers, industry, manufacturers, or an allergen bank.
> - The Internet offers a multitude of useful information databases.
> - "Difficult allergens" are those with a patch test concentration close to the irritancy threshold (i.e., emulsifiers, some biocides, and fragrance chemicals).

References

1. Diepgen TL, Andersen KE, Brandao FM, Bruze M, Bruynzeel DP, Frosch PJ, et al. Hand eczema classification: a cross-sectional, multicentre study of the aetiology and morphology of hand eczema. Br J Dermatol. 2009;160:353–8.
2. Cronin E. Clinical prediction of patch test results. Trans St Johns Hosp Dermatol Soc. 1972;58:153–62.
3. Cronin E. Clinical patterns of hand eczema in women. Contact Dermatitis. 1985;13:153–61.
4. Krautheim A, Lessmann H, Geier J. Patch testing with a patient's own materials handled at work. Chapter 82. In: Rustemeier T, Elsner P, John SM, Maibach HI, editors. Kanerva's occupational dermatology. Berlin/Heidelberg: Springer; 2012. p. 919–33.
5. Menne T, Dooms Goossens A, Wahlberg JE, White IR, Shaw S. How large a proportion of contact sensitivities are diagnosed with the European standard series? Contact Dermatitis. 1992;26:201–2.
6. Agner T, Andersen KE, Brandao FM, Bruze M, Bruynzeel DP, Frosch PJ, et al. Contact sensitization in hand eczema patients-relation to subdiagnosis, severity and quality of life: a multi-centre study. Contact Dermatitis. 2009;61:291–6.
7. de Groot AC. Patch testing, test concentrations and vehicles for 4350 chemicals. 3rd ed. Wapserveen: AC de Groot Publishing; 2008. p. 1–455.
8. Daecke CM, Schaller J, Goos M. Value of the patient's own test substances in epicutaneous testing. Hautarzt. 1994;45:292–8.
9. Slodownik D, Williams J, Frowen K, Palmer A, Matheson M, Nixon R. The additive value of patch testing with patient's own products at an occupational dermatology clinic. Contact Dermatitis. 2009;61:231–5.
10. Andersen KE. The allergen bank: the idea behind it and the preliminary results with it. Curr Probl Dermatol. 1995;22:1–7.

11. Andersen KE, Rastogi SC, Carlsen L. The allergen bank: a source of extra contact allergens for the dermatologist in practice. Acta Derm Venereol. 1996;76:136–40.
12. Goon ATJ, Bruze M, Zimerson E, Sorensen O, Goh CL, Koh DSQ, et al. Variation in allergen content over time of acrylates/methacrylates in patch test preparations. Br J Dermatol. 2011;164:116–24.
13. Mose KF, Andersen KE, Christensen LP. Stability of selected volatile contact allergens in different patch test chambers under different storage conditions. Contact Dermatitis. 2012;66: 72–179.
14. Gamboni SE, Simmons I, Palmer A, Nixon RL. Allergic contact dermatitis to indium in jewellery: diagnosis made possible through the use of the Contact Allergen Bank Australia. Australas J Dermatol. 2013;54:139–40.
15. Dall ABH, Andersen KE, Mortz CG. Targeted testing with diethylthiourea often reveals clinically relevant allergic contact dermatitis caused by neoprene rubber. Contact Dermatitis. 2012;67:89–93.
16. Mose AP, Frost S, Öhlund U, Andersen KE. Allergic contact dermatitis from octylisothiazolinone. Contact Dermatitis. 2013;69(1):49–52.
17. Christensson JB, Andersen KE, Bruze M, Johansen JD, Garcia-Bravo B, Gimenez-Arnau A, et al. An international multicenter study on the allergenic activity of air-oxidized R-limonene. Contact Dermatitis. 2013;68:214–23.
18. Christensson JB, Andersen KE, Bruze M, Johansen JD, Garcia-Bravo B, Gimenez-Arnau A, et al. Air-oxidized linalool – a frequent cause of fragrance contact allergy. Contact Dermatitis. 2012;67:247–59.

Occupational Allergic Contact Dermatitis: New Facets

7

An E. Goossens

Biocides, resins, rubber additives, drugs, and, to a minor extent, botanically derived materials and metals (particularly nickel) are gaining attention in the literature as occupational allergens.

7.1 Biocides

Isothiazolinone derivatives, biocides (preservatives) widely used in order to protect water-based products such as cosmetics, and household and industrial products have been increasingly reported as causes of occupational contact dermatitis. The lesions are often airborne induced and sometimes accompanied by respiratory and other systemic symptoms [1].

The mixture of methylchloroisothiazolinone (MCI) and methylisothiazolinone (MI) and, more recently, MI alone, which is a weaker allergen than MCI but equally sensitizing because of higher use concentrations, are used in cosmetics and, together with octyl- and benzisothiazolinone, also used in household and industrial products. Detergents and other cleansing products, even ironing water [2], cooling fluids [3], printing inks (data on file), glues (also for wallpaper) [4], and paints [5], are common sensitization sources. MI is actually causing an epidemic in Europe [6] and apparently also in the United States [7], mainly due to its presence in cosmetics and paints, in which the latter, together with epoxy resins, are notorious occupational allergens [5]. Moreover, sensitized consumers are at risk for developing severe airborne dermatitis when exposed to freshly painted walls. Figure 7.1 illustrates a hairdresser with hand dermatitis sensitized by MI-containing hair-care products and who, during several weeks, suffered from airborne dermatitis caused by contact with freshly painted walls that were releasing this biocide. Indeed, it has been shown

A.E. Goossens, RPharm, PhD
Department of Dermatology, Katholieke Universiteit Leuven,
Kapucijnenvoer 33, Leuven 3000, Belgium
e-mail: an.goossens@uzleuven.be

J.-M. Lachapelle et al. (eds.), *Patch Testing Tips*,
DOI 10.1007/978-3-642-45395-3_7, © Springer-Verlag Berlin Heidelberg 2014

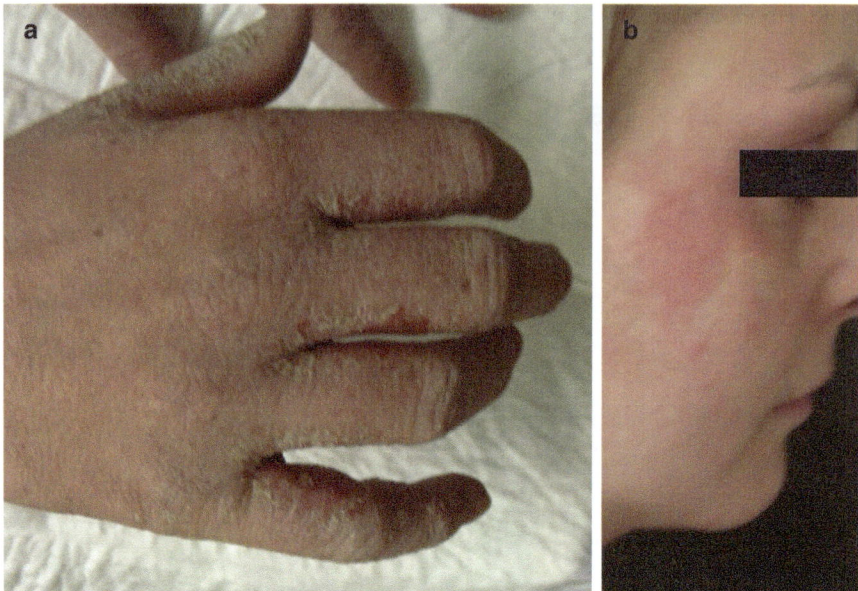

Fig. 7.1 (**a**) Severe hand dermatitis in a young female hairdresser sensitized by methylisothiazo-linone in hair-care products. (**b**) Airborne dermatitis in the same patient caused by freshly painted walls at home releasing this biocide

that the isothiazolinones' air concentrations may be released from paint for up to several weeks [8]; hence, abolition of symptoms by chemical allergen inactivation (using sodium bisulfite, also a notorious allergen) [9] or the use of preservative-free paints by alkalization to prevent microbial contamination [10] has been proposed.

Moreover, isothiazolinones are also being incorporated in other materials, such as benzisothiazolinone in medical vinyl gloves [11] and even in textiles (e.g., "sani-tized" sheets and mattress covers treated against house dust mites and insects). For example, the introduction of a new "biocide" in 2005 (with high concentrations of MCI/MI) in a Belgian factory (data on file) of such mattress covers resulted in several cases of airborne dermatitis and respiratory problems. Patch testing showed positive reactions to MCI/MI in 6 of 11 workers with skin complaints, 2 of whom also showed a positive reaction to octylisothiazolinone and 1 to benzisothiazoli-none, all of which were present in the biocide solutions. In the five other workers, the skin lesions were considered irritant. Four subjects also suffered from respiratory complaints.

In addition to the mixture MCI/MI at 100 ppm that often produces false-negative results, MI should also be tested in the baseline series, at 2,000 ppm (using a micro-pipette for application) that has recently been recommended [12].

Formaldehyde contact sensitivity, which was previously reported with a steady frequency in Europe, seems to have recently somewhat increased [13]. Occupational allergic contact dermatitis from formaldehyde releasers may occur in beauticians and hairdressers and other occupations and may occasionally be accompanied by

Fig. 7.2 Conjunctivitis and dermatitis in a mechanic in contact with polypropylene fibers preserved with 1, 3, 5-tris (2-hydroxyethyl)-hexahydrotriazine

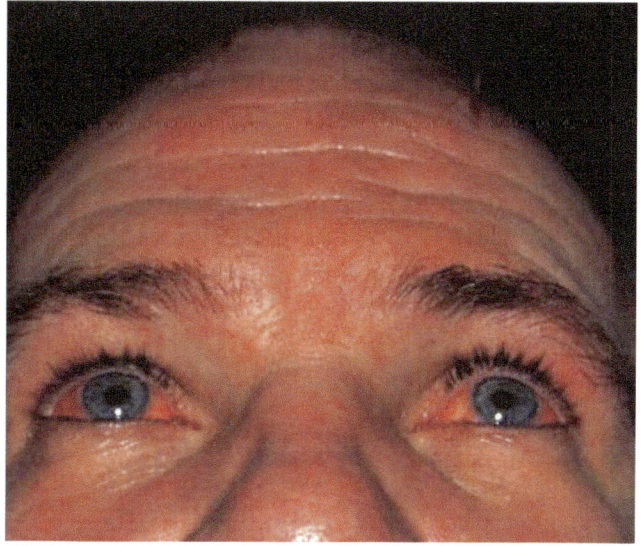

conjunctivitis and respiratory problems. Figure 7.2 shows a mechanic who suffered from dermatitis, conjunctivitis, and asthma due to contact with 1,3,5-tris (2-hydroxyethyl)-hexahydrotriazine used for preservation of polypropylene fibers [14].

Formaldehyde has also been detected in reusable polyvinyl chloride (PVC) and nitrile gloves [15]. Figure 7.3 shows a positive test to a formaldehyde-containing PVC glove that has caused hand dermatitis in a sensitized individual.

In addition to biocides, recently triphenyl phosphite, previously described in other occupational settings [16, 17], has also been identified as an allergen in PVC gloves [18, 19]. It is used as a stabilizer in many types of polymer, such as polyesters, polyethylene, PVC, polyurethane, and epoxy compounds, and in adhesives and coatings. It also provides increased heat resistance to the finished products as a flame retardant.

7.2 Resins

Resins are important sensitizers used in various domains and are often responsible for airborne immediate and delayed allergic reactions.

Acrylic resins are allergens in printing, glues, coatings, paints, and also nail cosmetics; the latter are an increasingly important source of contact allergy in beauticians (and hairdressers), and they may also be responsible for respiratory problems [20]. Fortunately, the occurrence of allergic contact dermatitis from acrylic resins (and also epoxy-acrylates) in dentists and dental technicians has diminished due to no-touch techniques. Nitrile gloves are said to be efficient in occupational acrylate allergy but need to be changed between procedures.

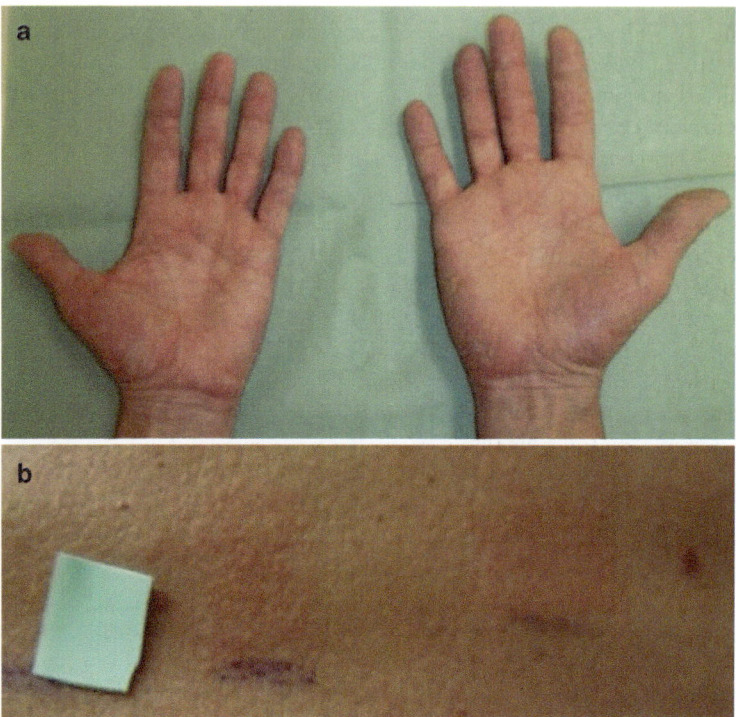

Fig. 7.3 (**a**) Hand dermatitis due to formaldehyde-containing PVC gloves. (**b**) Positive reactions to both the inner and outer side of the gloves

Since the test materials are instable due to evaporation [21], they should be kept in the freezer and applied immediately before patch testing (using plastic chambers)!

Epoxy resins based on diglycidyl ether of the bisphenol A type (present in the baseline series) have been known as allergens for many decades. Also, newer types, such as bisphenol F-based resins, are found. Epoxy resins are still widely used, for example, in hydraulic fluids [22], to impregnate fibers used in the aircraft industry, the manufacture of electronic circuits [23] and wind turbine rotor blades [24], but also in construction [25]; more recently, they have been identified as allergens in pipe lining [26]. Epoxy resins are also constituents of paints, in which they are the second most important allergens besides isothiazolinones [5]. Last but not least, as with other resins, testing with the materials contacted at work may be extremely valuable [27].

In contrast to their potential for being respiratory allergens, isocyanates (in polyurethanes)

have also been increasingly recognized as skin allergens in various domains, such as in the production of motor vehicles, in the electronics and paint industries, in construction work [28], in jewelry [29], and, lastly, in (epoxy-lacquered aluminum) heat exchangers [30]. However, in order to diagnose contact allergy to them, patch testing needs to be performed with the materials contacted at work as well as with diaminodiphenyl methane [31], a marker for isocyanate allergy (MDI) sensitivity. Indeed, the commercially available patch test materials have been found to be inadequate. They should also be kept in the freezer and applied immediately before patch testing.

7.3 Rubber Additives

So-called non-latex gloves are causing confusion among consumers since they may be free of latex proteins causing type I allergy, but "natural" rubber latex and "synthetic" latex-free rubber (also nitrile!) medical gloves do contain the same allergenic rubber additives.

Recently, the number of contact-allergic reactions to 1, 3-diphenylguanidine and carbamate derivatives has increased, with some of these patients also reacting to thiuram- derivatives, mercaptobenzothiazole, and cyclohexylthiophthalimide [32].

Synthetic rubber gloves probably contain higher amounts of rubber allergens in order to render them more elastic, and skin irritation due to antibacterial agents such as cetylpyridinium chloride (a quaternary ammonium compound) is followed by better skin penetration of the additives. The presence of these chemicals in gloves has been confirmed and is responsible for the recent increase in occupational contact dermatitis in surgical operating theater personnel [33].

7.4 Drugs

Drugs and their intermediates have been described as allergenic culprits in the chemical and pharmaceutical industries; however, allergic contact dermatitis in nurses from drugs administered to patients has become a frequent finding. Tetrazepam, in particular [34, 35], and other benzodiazepines (which, in contrast to systemic exposure, seem to cross-react following skin contact) are (mainly airborne) allergenic culprits in health-care workers (or relatives) crushing drug tablets for patients with difficulty swallowing [34, 35] (Fig. 7.4). In our experience, such patients often present with multiple positive reactions, also to non-related drugs; hence, patch testing with all contacted medicaments and possible cross-reacting molecules is indicated. Prevention by the use of crushing devices and protective measures (gloves and masks) should therefore be advised. Moreover, corticosteroid aerosols and particularly budesonide [36] may sensitize health-care workers and relatives in contact with the patients who are using them.

Moreover, antiseptics and disinfectants containing quaternary ammonium compounds such as didecyl dimethyl ammonium chloride are gaining importance as occupational immediate-type and delayed-type allergens in this profession [37, 38]. Even isopropanol may be an occupational sensitizer [39].

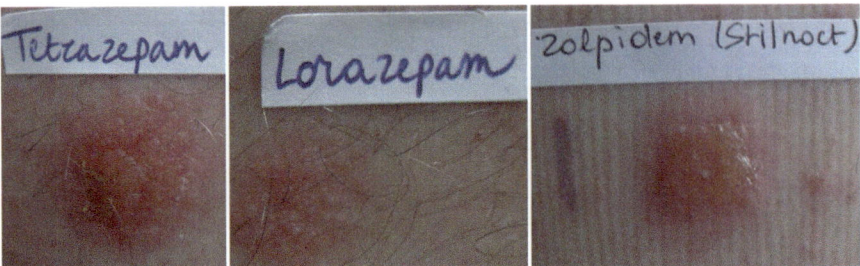

Fig. 7.4 Multiple positive reactions in a health-care worker who has suffered from severe airborne dermatitis when crushing drugs for disabled people

7.5 Botanically Derived Materials

There is growing interest in natural remedies, herbal products, and aromatherapy affecting beauticians and aromatherapists. Concomitant or cross-reactivity to multiple fragrance components is being observed, due to the common presence of air-oxidized terpenes [40] – for example, limonene [41] and linalool [42], which are definitely important allergens and should even be considered for addition to the baseline series.

Occupational immunologic contact urticaria (ICU) due to hydrolyzed proteins is also a potential hazard in beauticians and hairdressers; recently, high molecular weight hydrolyzed wheat proteins were demonstrated to have more allergenic than the hydrolysates having a lower molecular weight substances [43].

7.6 Metals

Recently, attention has been drawn to the potential role of nickel in coins for cashiers [44] and its release from the top and/or bottom surfaces of laptop computers as well as from computer mice [45]. With regard to a more exceptional allergen, rhodium was found to be an airborne cause of dermatitis in a jeweler (who also presented with respiratory symptoms) and a metal refinery worker [46].

Conclusion
Recent literature reports on occupationally induced skin lesions concern biocides, particularly isothiazolinones, and resins (i.e., epoxy, acrylates, and isocyanates, with painters being a high-risk profession in this regard); rubber additives, particularly carbamates and diphenylguanidine in medical "latex"-free synthetic rubber gloves; systemic drugs administered to patients in health-care personnel; botanically derived materials in aromatherapists and beauticians; and nickel as an allergen in cashiers and those involved in computer work. Particular attention should be given to the airborne nature of the allergens (both immediate and

delayed type) caused by components that are first released into the air (dust, droplets, and volatile substances) and then settle on the exposed skin [47]. Moreover, airborne contact dermatitis is occasionally associated with respiratory and also other systemic symptoms.

Practical Tips
- Biocides and resins, rubber additives, and systemically administered drugs are gaining attention as occupational allergen sources in painters and health-care workers, respectively.
- Isothiazolinones are allergenic culprits in various domains.
- Both occupational immediate- and delayed-type allergic reactions are frequently observed, and both low and high molecular weight molecules may be involved.
- Testing with materials contacted at work has an extra value.
- Particular attention should be given to airborne contact dermatitis and the association with respiratory and also other systemic symptoms.

References

1. Kaur-Knudsen D, Menné T, Carlsen BC. Systemic allergic dermatitis following airborne exposure to 1, 2-benzisothiazolin-3-one. Contact Dermatitis. 2012;67:310–2.
2. Hunter KJ, Shelley JC, Haworth AE. Airborne allergic contact dermatitis to methylchloroisothiazolinone/ methylisothiazolinone in ironing water. Contact Dermatitis. 2008;58:183–4.
3. Henriks-Eckerman M-L, Jolanki R, Suuronen K. Sensitizing ingredients in metalworking fluid (MWF) concentrations. Contact Dermatitis. 2008;58(suppl):51.
4. Fischer T, Bohlin S, Edling C, Rystedt I, Wieslander G. Skin disease and contact sensitivity in house painters using water-based paints, glues and putties. Contact Dermatitis. 1995;32:39–45.
5. Mose AP, Lundov MD, Zachariae C, Menné T, Veien NK, Laurberg G, et al. Occupational contact dermatitis in painters – an analysis of patch test data from the Danish Contact Dermatitis Group. Contact Dermatitis. 2012;67:293–7.
6. Gonçalo M, Goossens A. Whilst Rome burns: the epidemic of contact allergy to methylisothiazolinone (editorial). Contact Dermatitis. 2013;68:257–8.
7. Castanedo-Tardana M, Zug K. Methylisothiazolinone. Dermatitis. 2013;24:2–6.
8. Bohn S, Niederer M, Brehm K, Bircher AJ. Airborne contact dermatitis from methylchloroisothiazolinone in wall paint. Abolition of symptoms by chemical allergen inactivation. Contact Dermatitis. 2000;42:196–201.
9. Garcia-Gavín J, Parente J, Goossens A. Allergic contact dermatitis caused by sodium metabisulfite, a challenging allergen. A case series and literature review. Contact Dermatitis. 2012;67:62–9.
10. Braun-Falco M, Knott E, Huss-Marp J, Ring J, Hofmann H. Alkalization of wall paint prevents airborne contact dermatitis in patients with sensitization to isothiazolinones. Contact Dermatitis. 2008;59:129–31.
11. Aalto-Korte K, Ackermann L, Henriks-Eckerman M-L, Välimaa J, Reinikka-Railo H, Leppänen E, et al. 1, 2-Benzisothiazolin-3-one (BIT) in disposable polyvinyl chloride gloves for medical use. Contact Dermatitis. 2007;57:365–70.

12. Bruze M, Engfeldt M, Gonçalo M, et al. Recommendation to include methylisothiazolinone in the European baseline patch test series. On behalf of the ESCD and EECDRG. Contact Dermatitis. 2013;69:263–70.
13. Svedman C, Andersen KE, Brandão FM, Bruynzeel DP, Diepgen TL, Frosch PJ, et al. Follow-up of the monitored levels of preservative sensitivity in Europe. Overview of the years 2001–2008. Contact Dermatitis. 2012;67:306–20.
14. Rasschaert V, Goossens A. Conjunctivitis and bronchial asthma: symptoms of contact allergy to 1, 3, 5- tris (2-hydroxyethyl) – hexahydrotriazine (Grotan BK). Contact Dermatitis. 2002;47:116.
15. Pontén A. Formaldehyde in reusable protective gloves. Contact Dermatitis. 2006;54:268–71.
16. Suuronen K, Pesonen M, Henriks-Eckerman M-L, Aalto-Korte K. Triphenyl phosphite, a new allergen in polyvinylchloride gloves. Contact Dermatitis. 2013;68:42–9.
17. Vandevenne A, Ghys K, Dahlin J, Pontén A, Kerre S. Allergic contact dermatitis caused by triphenyl phosphite in poly (vinyl chloride) gloves. Contact Dermatitis. 2013;68:181–2.
18. Sasseville D, Moreau L. Allergic contact dermatitis from triphenyl phosphite. Contact Dermatitis. 2005;52:163–4.
19. O'Driscoll JB, Marcus R, Beck MH. Occupational allergic contact dermatitis from triphenyl phosphite. Contact Dermatitis. 1989;20:392–3.
20. Jurado-Palomo J, Caballero T, Fernández-Nieto M, Quirce S. Occupational asthma caused by artificial cyanoacrylate fingernails. Ann Allergy Asthma Immunol. 2009;102:440–1.
21. Mose KF, Andersen KE, Christensen LP. Stability of selected volatile contact allergens in different patch test chambers under different storage conditions. Contact Dermatitis. 2012;66: 172–9.
22. Maibach HI, Mathias CT. Allergic contact dermatitis from cycloaliphatic epoxide in jet aviation hydraulic fluid. Contact Dermatitis. 2001;45:56.
23. Wenk KS, Ehrlich A. Allergic contact dermatitis from epoxy resin in solder mask coating in an individual working with printed circuit boards. Dermatitis. 2010;21:288–90.
24. Pontén A, Carstensen O, Rasmussens K, Gruvberger B, Isaksson M, Bruze M. Epoxy-based production of wind turbine rotor blades: occupational contact allergies. Dermatitis. 2004;15:33–40.
25. Geier J, Lessmann H, Reinecke S. Occupational airborne allergic contact dermatitis in a concrete repair worker. Contact Dermatitis. 2009;60:50–1.
26. Berglind IA, Lind M-L, Lidén C. Epoxy pipe relining – an emerging contact allergy risk for workers. Contact Dermatitis. 2012;67:59–65.
27. Houle MC, Holness DL, DeKoven J, Skotnicki S. Additive value of patch testing custom epoxy materials from the workplace at the Occupational Disease Specialty Clinic in Toronto. Dermatitis. 2012;23:214–9.
28. Aalto-Korte K, Suuronen K, Kuuliala O, Henriks-Eckerman ML, Jolanki R. Occupational contact allergy to monomeric isocyanates. Contact Dermatitis. 2012;67:78–88.
29. Nguyen R, Lee A. Allergic contact dermatitis caused by isocyanates in resin jewellery. Contact Dermatitis. 2012;67:56–7.
30. Engfeldt M, Isaksson M, Zimerson E, Bruze M. Several cases of work-related allergic contact dermatitis caused by isocyanates at a company manufacturing heat exchangers. Contact Dermatitis. 2013;68:175–80.
31. Engfeldt M, Goossens A, Isaksson M, Zimerson E, Bruze M. The outcome of 9 years of consecutive patch testing with 4,4'-diaminodiphenylmethane and 4,4'-diphenylmethane diisocyanate. Contact Dermatitis. 2013;68:98–102.
32. Baeck M, Cawet B, Tennstedt D, Goossens A. Allergic contact dermatitis from latex (natural rubber) – free gloves in healthcare workers. Contact Dermatitis. 2013;68:54–5.
33. Pontén A, Hamnerius N, Bruze M, Hansson C, Persson C, Svedman C, et al. Occupational allergic contact dermatitis caused by sterile non-latex protective gloves: clinical investigation and chemical analyses. Contact Dermatitis. 2013;68:103–10.
34. Vander Hulst K, Kerre S, Goossens A. Occupational allergic contact dermatitis from tetrazepam in nurses. Contact Dermatitis. 2010;62:303–8.

35. Landeck L, Skudlik C, John SM. Airborne contact dermatitis to tetrazepam in geriatric nurses-a report of 10 cases. Eur J Dermatol. 2012;26:680–4.
36. Baeck M, Goossens A. Patients with airborne sensitization/contact dermatitis from budesonide-containing aerosols 'by proxy'Contact. Dermatitis. 2009;61:1–8.
37. Houtappel M, Bruijnzeel-Koomen CAFM, Röckmann H. Immediate-type allergy by occupational exposure to didecyl dimethyl ammonium chloride. Contact Dermatitis. 2008;59:116–7.
38. Dejobert Y, Delaporte E, Piette F, et al. Contact dermatitis from didecyldimethylammonium chloride in detergent-disinfectants used in hospital: 5 cases. Contact Dermatitis. 2002; 46(suppl):60.
39. Garcia-Gavin J, Lissens R, Timmermans A, Goossens A. Allergic contact dermatitis caused by isopropyl alcohol: a missed allergen? Contact Dermatitis. 2011;65:101–6.
40. Paulsen E, Andersen KE. Colophonium and compositae mix as markers of fragrance allergy: cross-reactivity between fragrance terpenes, colophonium and compositae plant extracts. Contact Dermatitis. 2005;53:285–91.
41. Brared Christensson J, Andersen KE, Bruze M, Johansen JD, Garcia-Bravo B, Giménez-Arnau A, et al. An international multicentre study on the allergenic activity of air-oxidized R-limonene. Contact Dermatitis. 2013;68:214–23.
42. Brared Christensson J, Andersen KE, Bruze M, Johansen JD, Garcia-Bravo B, Gimenez Arnau A, et al. Air-oxidized linalool – a frequent cause of fragrance contact allergy. Contact Dermatitis. 2012;67:247–59.
43. Chinuki Y, Takahashi H, Dekio I, Kaneko S, Tokuda R, Nagao M, et al. Higher allergenicity of high molecular weight hydrolysed wheat protein in cosmetics for percutaneous sensitization. Contact Dermatitis. 2013;68:86–93.
44. Thyssen JP, Gawkrodger DJ, White IR, Julander A, Menné T, Lidén C. Coin exposure may cause allergic nickel dermatitis: a review. Contact Dermatitis. 2013;68:3–14.
45. Jensen P, Jellesen MS, Møller P, Johansen JD, Lidén C, Menné T, et al. Nickel may be released from laptop computers. Contact Dermatitis. 2012;67:384–5.
46. Goossens A, Cattaert N, Nemery B, Boey L, De Graef E. Occupational allergic contact dermatitis caused by rhodium solutions. Contact Dermatitis. 2011;64:158–61.
47. Swinnen I, Goossens A. An update on airborne contact dermatitis: 2007–2011. Contact Dermatitis. 2013;68:232–8.

Patch Testing and Atopic Eczema

8

Thomas L. Diepgen

8.1 Introduction

Atopic eczema (AE) is a common, chronically relapsing, inflammatory skin disease, clinically characterized by typically distributed eczematous lesions, dry skin, intense pruritus, and a wide variety of pathophysiologic aspects [1]. The clinical phenotype that characterizes AE is the product of interactions between susceptibility genes, the environment, defective skin barrier function, and immunologic responses [2].

AE is often associated with sensitizations against immediate-type allergens (type I allergy), like grass pollen, house dust mites, dander, food allergens, and others. Most common are sensitizations against aero- and food allergens. However, allergic sensitization (type I allergy) is neither a prerequisite for childhood eczema nor a uniform cause of AE. Patients with AE often develop allergic rhino-conjunctivitis and/or allergic asthma later in life, but there also exists a nonallergic subtype of AE that is defined by low IgE serum levels (<150 kU/l) and no detectable sensitizations against aero- and food allergens. This type is also called intrinsic AE.

In contrast to type I allergy, there is an ongoing debate about the relationship between delayed-type contact allergy (type IV allergy) and AE and on the issue of whether patients with AE are more or less prone to (occupational) delayed-type contact allergy.

By reading different studies about the relationship between delayed-type contact allergy and AE, an important question is whether the cases the publication deals with really have AE. In other words, was AE correctly assessed, without observer bias? A reliable diagnosis of AE is always important when patch testing is done, since AE is also part of the MOAHLFA index, which is an established tool to compare the important characteristics of patients of different patch test clinics [3]. The

T.L. Diepgen, MD, PhD
Department of Social Medicine, University Hospital Heidelberg,
Thibautstrasse 3, Heidelberg, Baden-Württemberg 69115, Germany
e-mail: thomas.diepgen@med.uni-heidelberg.de

J.-M. Lachapelle et al. (eds.), *Patch Testing Tips*,
DOI 10.1007/978-3-642-45395-3_8, © Springer-Verlag Berlin Heidelberg 2014

MOAHLFA index consists of the following items to describe the profile of the tested population: "M" men, "O" occupational dermatitis, "A" atopic eczema, "H" hand eczema, "L" leg dermatitis, "F" face dermatitis, and "A" age over 40 years. It is obvious that it is important to establish a standardized diagnosis of AE and atopic skin diathesis (ASD) when doing patch testing.

Therefore, in this chapter the following aspects of patch testing and AE are highlighted: how to establish a clear diagnosis of AE and ASD, the relationship between AE and hand eczema, and what can we learn from studies comparing patch test results in AE and non-AE.

8.2   How to Establish the Diagnosis of AE and Atopic Skin Diathesis

Until now there exist no laboratory markers for the diagnosis of AE, and the diagnosis is based on clinical criteria. In most cases, the diagnosis of AE can easily be made based on (family) history and clinical examination. However, to establish a firm diagnosis of AE, all patients have to be assessed by a combination of detailed clinical examination and anamnestic questions [4–7]. These criteria are considered important parameters to diagnose AE and were recently used to stratify AE and evaluated in different types of the course of AE [8].

AE often starts during the first year of life; this form is classified as the "early type of onset" of AE [9]. However, in some patients AE is not present during childhood but starts or relapses later in life (i.e., after 20 years of age) [10]. In a recent study, it could be demonstrated that the natural course of AE can be divided into subgroups that display different clinical features [8]. This study supports the assumption of a broad heterogeneity of AE in adolescence and adulthood and emphasizes the future need for careful stratification of patients with AE.

Lammintausta [11] introduced the term atopic skin diatheses as a useful definition of the skin condition that might be involved in the development of hand eczema. This condition was defined as (1) dry skin, (2) a history of low pruritus threshold for two of three nonspecific irritants (sweat, dust, rough material), (3) white dermographism, and (4) facial pallor/infraorbital darkening. This ASD significantly increased the risk of hand eczema among employees engaged in wet work.

In order to establish a diagnostic score for AE and ASD, basic and minor features of AE were evaluated systematically in established cases of AE and in subjects randomly collected from the Caucasian population of young adults in a prospective study [6]. Anamnestic and clinical atopic basic and minor features were investigated in all test subjects by two investigators to obtain a good interobserver agreement. Based on statistical modeling methods, a diagnostic scoring system was constructed, based on anamnestic and clinical features without laboratory investigations (Table 8.1). The presence of an itching flexural dermatitis was not included since this was the selection base. For practical use, every atopic feature obtained a value between 1 and 3 points according to its statistical significance. Based on this scoring

Table 8.1 Criteria of atopic skin diathesis (ASD)

	Points
Family history of atopy (1st-degree relatives)	
Eczema	2
Respiratory atopy	1
Personal history of atopy	
Flexural eczema	
Allergic rhinitis	1
Allergic asthma	1
Cradle cap	1
Itch when sweating	3
Intolerance to wool	3
Intolerance to metal	1
Photophobia	1
Minor manifestations of AE	
Xerosis	3
Ear rhagades	2
Dyshidrosis	2
Pityriasis alba	2
Atopic foot/pulpitis sicca	2
Nipple eczema	2
Perlèche	1
Atopic stigmata	
Atopic palms	2
Hertoghe sign	2
Dirty neck	2
Keratosis pilaris	1
White dermographism	3
Acrocyanosis	1

Adapted from [5, 6]
Individuals with at least 10 points have an ASD; between 7 and 9 points, ASD is suspected

system, patients with more than 10 points should be considered to have ASD; patients with more than 6 points are suspected of having ASD.

In many cases, the diagnosis of atopic background must rest on clinical features while an absolute marker for AE awaits recognition. Therefore, it is important to examine the whole body carefully for minimal eczematous lesions at typical locations such as the neck, the flexural area of the elbow and knee, dorsa of the feet, ear rhagades, etc.

8.3 AE and Atopic Hand Eczema

It is generally agreed that AE is characterized by a genetic predisposition to an impaired skin barrier and a reduced resistance to irritants and that consequently individuals with a history of or with current AE have a tendency to develop irritant contact dermatitis (ICD) located mainly on the hands. The genetic predisposition to an impaired barrier, for example, caused by loss-of-function mutations in the

Table 8.2 Characteristics of atopic hand eczema

Atopic hand eczema
Etiopathogenesis
Result of atopic eczema or atopic skin diathesis
Rarely also protein contact dermatitis
Frequently unrelated to occupation
Initial manifestation, transient or exacerbation by occupational toxins
Location
Often involves the backs of the hands as in irritant eczema
Involvement of the nails is common
Involvement of the flexor surfaces of the wrists is common, lichenification
Involvement of the "snuff box" through poorly bordered lichenified lesions
Involvement of other parts of the body (neck, flexure surfaces, dorsal aspects of the feet)
Morphology
Blistering is common (acro-vesicular morphology) palmar and interdigital
Lichenification (backs of the hands, flexor surfaces of wrists)
Scaling, rhagades (fingertips)
Nummular lesions (backs of hands, usually poorly bordered) possible

filaggrin gene, which are present in about one-third of Caucasian patients with AE, was identified as another potential risk factor for severe course of AE [12, 13].

In adults, the most common location of AE is the hands, and AE is a well-known risk factor influencing the course and prognosis of hand eczema [14].

The clinical pattern is dry, scaly, and fissuring skin at the dorsum of the hand with a tendency to lichenification (Table 8.2). In chronic cases, even a short direct skin contact to mild irritants such as water or wet work will induce a relapse of the inflammatory skin disease. It is most often impossible to distinguish between ICD on an atopic base caused by work-related exogenous factors and an atopic hand eczema mainly caused by endogenous factors. A typical pattern for the atopic hand eczema is the involvement of eczematous lesions at the wrist, in contrast to an ICD, where this location is unusual.

There is consensus that exposure to irritants precipitates or aggravates hand eczema in individuals with a history of AE [14, 15]. Usually, atopy or AE is considered as a "risk factor" for hand eczema. However, it is more logical to look at AE as an effect modifier, i.e., the question of what extent the presence of AE will elicit more skin reactions (hand eczema) from occupational exposure. In contrast to AE or "skin atopy," there is sufficient evidence that mucosal atopy, without skin manifestations, is not associated with increased risk of ICD [14, 16].

8.4   AE and Contact Allergy

There has been much debate on the issue of whether patients with AE develop more or less frequent contact allergy, and the literature on the relationship between AE and cutaneous delayed-type hypersensitivity is inclusive. Because AE patients differ from non-AE patients in immunologic responses and are harder to experimentally sensitize to the nonprotein allergens, patch test responses to commercially available patch test series may differ in AE patients. Some studies argue that there may be a slightly decreased risk; at least a "classical" type IV contact allergy to common sensitizers does not seem to be more prevalent among atopics. Some authors have claimed a decreased cell-mediated immunity among atopic individuals, which would lead to observations of decreased rates of allergic contact dermatitis (ACD).

On the other hand, AE patients often have an impaired barrier function, and one can argue that allergens can penetrate easier through the epidermal barrier and more frequently the induction of sensitization can be expected. It is also known that exposure to irritants can trigger sensitization to delayed-type contact allergens. Patients with AE are at high risk to develop ICD in many high-risk professions, and one could expect that therefore they also have a higher risk for contact allergy and ACD. Another point to consider is that AE patients have a higher exposure to emollients, topical corticosteroids, and antiseptics than nonatopics, especially since some of the used ingredients are well-known sensitizers. The combination of impaired barrier function and higher exposure would result in higher prevalence rates to at least some contact allergens. Looking at AE as a disease with many predisposing, precipitating, and perpetuating factors, it is obvious that exogenous factors like irritants and allergens can precipitate and perpetuate.

With respect to type I (IgE-mediated) contact urticarial reactions, which can develop into hand eczema, the situation is quite clear: immediate-type contact reactions to latex (gloves used by health-care personnel) or alpha-amylase (yeast used by bakers) or food proteins are much more common among atopics [17, 18]. The clinical result is also called protein contact dermatitis.

What can we learn from recent patch test studies in AE and non-AE patients? In a recent study from the United States, a total of 2,305 patients underwent patch testing to the NACDG (North American Contact Dermatitis Group) standard screening series. The incidence of positive patch test reaction among patients with AE ($n = 297$) and without AE ($n = 2,008$) was assessed [19]. Compared with nonatopic patients, those with AE were statistically more likely to have positive patch tests. AE was associated with contact hypersensitivity to nickel, cobalt, and chromium, but was not associated with contact sensitization to fragrances. In another recent study from the United States, the overall number of positive patch test results did not differ significantly in AE patients ($n = 146$) versus non-AE patients ($n = 1,003$) [20]. In this study there was no significant increase in nickel sensitivity, but there was no significant trend toward an increased number of positive patch test reactions to tixocortol pivalate, compositae mix, and propylene glycol in AE patients.

Also in an occupational setting, AE patients seem to develop at least as much contact allergy as nonatopics. This is supported by data from a study among hairdressers (Table 8.3): even in this group of people, who are heavily exposed to occupational allergens, there are no significant differences in sensitization rates between those with atopic manifestations on the skin and nonatopics. This is in agreement with a study of 143 hairdressers with hand eczema in the United Kingdom: no significant difference was found between the eczematous atopics, mucous membrane

Table 8.3 Type IV contact allergy and atopic skin diathesis among hairdressers with notified occupational contact dermatitis in North Bavaria, Germany

	Atopic skin diathesis ($n=215$)	Nonatopics ($n=312$)
Occupational allergens		
Glyceryl monothioglycolate	48 %	54 %
p-Phenylenediamine	28 %	30 %
Ammonium persulfate	22 %	26 %
Nonoccupational allergens		
Nickel sulfate	49 %	45 %
Balsam of Peru	2 %	4 %

According to Diepgen, personal communication

atopics, and nonatopics in their capacity to be sensitized to hairdressing allergens or to nickel [21].

We recently assessed patients with notified occupational skin disease in the federal office for environmental and occupational protection in Saarbrücken, Germany, from 2000 to 2012. AE was diagnosed in 384 patients (22 %) out of a total of 1,772 cases. At least one contact allergy was diagnosed in 36 % of the AE patients ($n=384$) and in 32 % of the nonatopic patients ($n=1,388$). This study again demonstrates that contact allergy is at least as frequent in AE patients as it is in nonatopic patients with notified OSD.

How is the situation in the normal population? We conducted a large European survey to evaluate the frequency of contact allergies in the general population [22]. A random sample from the general population, aged 18–74 years, was selected in six European areas (Sweden, the Netherlands, Germany [two sites], Italy, Portugal); 12,377 subjects were interviewed and a random sample ($n=3,119$) patch tested to True test panel 1, 2, and 3. A positive patch test reaction (at least a "+" reaction) was considered as a proxy for contact allergy. The lifetime prevalence rate of AE was 7.6 %. The prevalence rate of at least one positive patch test reaction (contact allergy) to at least one of the tested allergens in True test panel 1–3 was 30.3 % in AE and 24.7 % in non-AE. Individuals with a personal history of AE had no increased or decreased risk of contact allergy to at least one of the tested allergens (OR 1.0, 95 % CI 0.7–1.4). There was no significant increase in nickel contact allergy (OR 0.9, 95 % CI 0.6–1.4) or fragrance contact allergy (OR 1.1, 95 % CI 0.6–2.0).

In conclusion, patients with AE should be patch tested when indicated because they also develop contact allergic sensitization to a significant degree. Patch testing often adds valuable information about contact allergy in these patients.

8.5   Attributable Risk for Occupational Skin Diseases

From a prevention point of view, it is important to quantify the proportion of OSD in the working population that may be attributable to AE or ASD. The attributable risk (AR) is the adequate measure to estimate this proportion. Assuming that ASD

Table 8.4 Odds ratio (OR) and attributable risk (AR) in cases with notified occupational skin disease (OSD) for the risk factor of atopic skin diathesis (ASD) in selected professions

Occupational group	Insured persons	Incidence rate of cases with an OSD (95 %CI)	$OR_{(ASD)}$ (95 %CI)	$AR_{(ASD)}$[a] (95%CI)
	(Average number of employees over 10 years)	(Per 10,000 workers per year)	$p_{(ASD)} = 20$ %	
Pastry cooks	2,188	20.6 (14.6–26.6)	7.0 (3.8–12.8)	53.3 (35.7–70.8)
Bakers	4,221	33.2 (27.8–38.6)	5.8 (4.1–8.2)	47.3 (37.2–57.4)
Florists	1,548	23.9 (16.3–31.5)	5.0 (2.6–9.6)	43.1 (23.2–63.1)
Health-care workers	65,731	7.3 (6.7–8.0)	4.0 (3.4–4.8)	37.4 (31.8–43.0)
Cooks	17,007	6.6 (5.4–7.8)	3.7 (2.6–5.4)	34.9 (23.4–46.4)
Dental technicians	2,508	10.8 (6.7–14.9)	3.3 (1.5–7.0)	30.8 (7.4–54.2)
Locksmiths and automobile mechanics	54,827	2.2 (1.8–2.6)	3.2 (2.2–4.6)	30.7 (19.6–41.9)
Mechanics	6,688	6.0 (4.1–7.9)	2.7 (1.4–5.1)	25.1 (6.1–44.1)
Food-processing industry and butchers	15,836	2.9 (2.1–3.7)	2.6 (1.4–4.7)	24.0 (6.3–41.6)
Hairdressers and barbers	8,792	97.4 (91.2–103.6)	2.3 (1.9–2.6)	18.9 (14.9–22.9)

Adapted from [23]
[a]AR as percent and provided if OR ≥ 1

can be monitored and a work-related manifestation as AE or ICD would be preventable in those individuals in high-risk professions, public health authorities should have a genuine interest in estimating the proportion of work-related skin diseases that could be prevented.

Therefore, we determined the odds ratio (OR) and attributable risk (AR) of OSDs in the working population due to ASD and assessed the potential for preventive interventions in different professions in North Bavaria [23]. Based on about 460,000 employees, the annual incidence rate of notified OSD was 6.7 cases per 10,000 workers (95 % CI 6.5–6.9). Assuming that the prevalence of ASD is 20 % in the general population, the risk of developing a notified occupational skin disease is 240 % increased in persons with an ASD compared to individuals without (OR 2.4; 95 % CI 2.2–2.6). The AR of ASD was calculated to be 21.6 (AR 21.6; 95 % CI 19.4–23.7); that means that 21.6 %, or at least one-fifth, of these OSDs could have been prevented if ASD among the working population could be monitored. Clearly, AR depends on ASD prevalence in the total population. Assuming, for example, 10 % or 30 % ASD in the total population, the average AR would increase to 30.3 % (95 % CI 28.4–32.2) or decrease to 10.3 (95 % CI 7.9–12.7), respectively.

The professions with the ten highest AR for ASD are presented in Table 8.4. Our findings illustrate the potential impact of ASD on OSDs in the context of preventive strategies, primarily in food preparation workers (pastry cooks, bakers, cooks), florists, and health-care workers.

Practical Tips

- Patients with AE should be patch tested when indicated because they also develop contact allergic sensitization to a significant degree.
- Patch testing often adds valuable information about contact allergy in these patients.
- A reliable diagnosis of AE is important whenever patch testing is done. To establish a firm diagnosis of AE, all patients have to be assessed by a combination of detailed clinical examination and anamnestic questions.
- Allergic contact dermatitis is not more common in AE; however, contact allergy is at least as common in AE patients as in non-AE patients.
- Occupational contact urticaria is more common in atopics.
- Occupational irritants precipitate AE and patients with AE are at risk of developing irritant hand eczema.
- Respiratory atopy without ASD is not a risk factor for hand eczema and allergic contact dermatitis.
- AE is probably an effect modifier for occupational exposure.

References

1. Diepgen TL. Occupational skin disease data in Europe. Int Arch Occup Environ Health. 2003;76:331–8.
2. Leung DY, Boguniewicz M, Howell MD, Nomura I, Hamid QA. New insights into atopic dermatitis. J Clin Invest. 2004;113:651–7.
3. Smith HR, Wakelin SH, McFadden JP, Rycroft RJ, White IR. A 15-year review of our MOAHLFA index. Contact Dermatitis. 1999;40:227–8.
4. Hanifin J, Rajka G. Diagnostic features of atopic eczema. Acta Derm Venereol. 1980;92:44–7.
5. Diepgen TL, Fartasch M, Hornstein OP. Evaluation and relevance of atopic basic and minor features in patients with atopic dermatitis and in the general population. Acta Derm Venereol Suppl (Stockh). 1989;144:50–4.
6. Diepgen TL, Sauerbrei W, Fartasch M. Development and validation of diagnostic scores for atopic dermatitis incorporating criteria of data quality and practical usefulness. J Clin Epidemiol. 1996;49:1031–8.
7. Williams HC, Burney PG, Hay RJ, Archer CB, Shipley MJ, Hunter JJ, et al. The U.K. working party's diagnostic criteria for atopic dermatitis. I. Derivation of a minimum set of discriminators for atopic dermatitis. Br J Dermatol. 1994;131:383–96.
8. Garmhausen D, Hagemann T, Bieber T, Dimitriou I, Fimmers R, Diepgen T, Novak N. Characterization of different courses of atopic dermatitis in adolescent and adult patients. Allergy. 2013;68:498–506.
9. Bieber T. Atopic dermatitis. N Engl J Med. 2008;358:1483–94.
10. Wuthrich B. Atopic neurodermatitis. Wien Med Wochenschr. 1989;139:156–65.
11. Lammintausta K. Risk factors for hand dermatitis in wet work. Academic dissertation, Turku; 1982.
12. Kezic S, O'Regan GM, Yau N, Sandilands A, Chen H, Campbell LE, et al. Levels of filaggrin degradation products are influenced by both filaggrin genotype and atopic dermatitis severity. Allergy. 2011;66:934–40.

13. Thyssen JP, Linneberg A, Johansen JD, Carlsen BC, Zachariae C, Meldgaard M, et al. Atopic diseases by filaggrin mutations and birth year. Allergy. 2012;67:705–8.
14. Rystedt I. Hand eczema in patients with history of atopic manifestations in childhood. Acta Derm Venereol (Stockh). 1985;65:305–12.
15. Meding B, Swanbeck G. Predictive factors for hand eczema. Contact Dermatitis. 1990;23:154–61.
16. Majoie IML, von Blomberg BME, Bruynzeel DP. Development of hand eczema in junior hairdressers: an 8-year follow-up study. Contact Dermatitis. 1996;34:243–7.
17. Rycroft RJG. Occupational contact dermatitis. In: Rycroft RJG, Menné T, Frosch PJ, Benezra C, editors. Textbook of contact dermatitis. 2nd ed. Berlin: Springer; 1995. p. 343–400.
18. Lahti A. Immediate contact reactions. In: Rycroft RJG, Menné T, Frosch PJ, Benezra C, editors. Textbook of contact dermatitis. 2nd ed. Berlin: Springer; 1995. p. 62–74.
19. Malajian D, Belsito DV. Cutaneous delayed-type hypersensitivity in patients with atopic dermatitis. J Am Acad Dermatol. 2013;69:232–7.
20. Nedorost ST, Cooper KD. The role of patch testing for chemical and protein allergens in atopic dermatitis. Curr Allergy Asthma Rep. 2001;1:323–8.
21. Sutthipisal N, McFadden JP, Cronin E. Sensitization in atopic and non-atopic hairdressers with hand eczema. Contact Dermatitis. 1993;29:206–9.
22. Rossi M, Coenraads PJ, Diepgen T, Svensson Å, Elsner P, Gonçalo M, et al. Design and feasibility of an international study assessing the prevalence of contact allergy to fragrances in the general population: the European Dermato-Epidemiology Network Fragrance Study. Dermatology. 2010;221:267–75.
23. Dickel H, Bruckner TM, Schmidt A, Diepgen TL. Impact of atopic skin diathesis on occupational skin disease incidence in a working population. J Invest Dermatol. 2003;121:37–40.

Occupational Airborne Contact Dermatitis: A Realm for Specific Diagnostic Procedures and Tips

Jean-Marie Lachapelle

9.1 Introduction

Most patients consulting in occupational dermatology are referred to as irritant or allergic contact dermatitis cases; conceptually, the term "contact dermatitis" implies a direct contact of the skin with the offending (liquid and/or solid) agents. It is not surprising that in this respect, hand dermatitis is the major complaint; this is due to a direct manipulation – at work – of thousands of different products. It is clear that other skin sites can also be affected, either directly or indirectly (transfer of chemicals by hands).

Apart from this "familiar landscape," the occurrence of occupational airborne dermatoses, that is, due to agents carried by or through the air, has been underestimated in the past.

In the 1980s, more attention was paid to the problem, after the publication of two review articles [1, 2]. In 2007, Santos and Goossens [3] updated in a review paper (2001–2006) a list of offending agents able to provoke airborne contact dermatitis. This review has been completed in full detail very recently, to include new chemicals involved in the occurrence of airborne contact dermatitis (ABCD) [4].

They consider that the figures are underestimated for two main reasons: (1) many original cases are never published, and (2) in some papers, the term "airborne" does not appear in the keywords and the publications are therefore omitted in general reviews. Today, each year brings new observations, coming from various parts of the world. These publications reflect the diversity of problems encountered, in relation to new chemicals and/or modified technical procedures. A better knowledge of occupational airborne dermatoses has practical implications, in terms of diagnosis, treatment, and prevention. There is a clear distinction to be made between airborne dermatoses and the

J.-M. Lachapelle, MD, PhD
Department of Dermatology, Catholic University of Louvain,
Cliniques Universitaires Saint-Luc,
10, Avenue Hippocrate, Brussels B-1200, Belgium
e-mail: jean-marie.lachapelle@uclouvain.be

J.-M. Lachapelle et al. (eds.), *Patch Testing Tips*,
DOI 10.1007/978-3-642-45395-3_9, © Springer-Verlag Berlin Heidelberg 2014

"sick building syndrome" (SBS); the latter refers to epidemics of subjective symptoms (itching or burning sensations) without any clinically visible signs, which occur in the work environment. This situation can be related, for instance, to a low relative humidity rate in the air but may also represent a mass psychogenic illness.

This chapter is focused on occupational ABCD but, conceptually, can of course be extended to other environmental nonoccupational cases of ABCD [4].

9.2   A Short Review of Airborne Offending Agents

It is common to consider three types of airborne offending agents.

9.2.1   Fibers

Different types of fibers can be implied [5, 6]. The most classical example is fiber-glass. Other examples include rockwool, carbon fibers, plastic materials such as polypropylene fibers, etc. Fibers can be chemically inert and provoke only mechanical trauma to the skin. Carbon fiber dermatitis and most cases of fiberglass dermatitis are good examples of this condition. On the other hand, some fibers can produce allergic reactions, such as epoxy-coated fiberglass.

9.2.2   Dust Particles

Dust is ubiquitous in the work environment. Dust particles are transported by air; they can accumulate on the surface of the skin, in a visible way or not. Like fibers, some dust particles are chemically inert but can provoke mechanical (frictional) injury to the skin, whereas others do contain chemicals that are dissolved by the sweat; according to their nature, these chemicals are responsible for several types of skin reactions.

9.2.3   Sprays

Water- or other liquid-based products moving in a mass of dispersed droplets represent an important source of airborne offending agents. Any of numerous commercial products, including paints, cosmetics, and insecticides that are dispensed from containers in this manner, are good examples. Skin reactions are multifaceted: irritant, eczematous, urticarial, or combined.

9.2.4   Vapors and Gases

Vapor is defined as barely visible or cloudy diffused matter, such as mist, fumes, or smoke, suspended in the air. Gas has a more restricted meaning. Vapors and gases may be, like sprays, irritant, allergenic, or both.

Table 9.1 Classification of occupational airborne contact dermatoses

1	Irritant ABCD (frictional and/or chemical)
2	Allergic ABCD
3	Phototoxic (photo irritant) ABCD
4	Photoallergic ABCD
5	Airborne (immunological and/or non-immunological) contact urticaria
6	Exacerbation of extrinsic atopic dermatitis by aeroallergens("face and neck dermatitis")
7	The sick building syndrome

Fig. 9.1 The usual topography of different types of ABCD

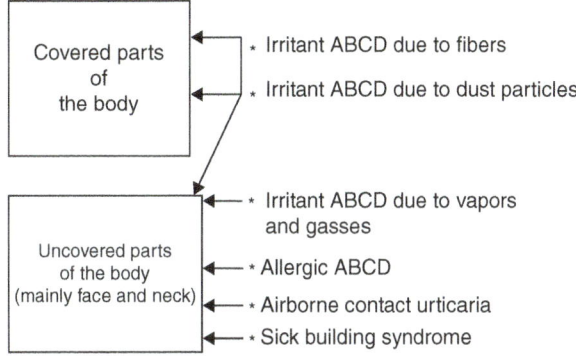

9.3   Classification of Occupational Airborne Contact Dermatoses

A classification of occupational airborne contact dermatoses is presented in Table 9.1.

9.4   Topography of Lesions in the Various Types of ABCD

The topography of skin lesions in the various types of ABCD is an important clue for a preliminary approach to the diagnosis (Fig. 9.1) [7].

This general profile of localization is indicative, but, in some rare cases, overlapping is to be considered.

9.5   Clinical Signs and Symptoms of the Various Types of ABCD

9.5.1   ABCD due to Fibers

The prototype is fiberglass dermatitis, by far the most frequent condition (Fig. 9.2). It is still a very important problem in occupational dermatology, as mentioned in recent papers [8, 9]. A very important contribution has been made about the configuration of glass fibers by scanning electron microscopy [10].

Fig. 9.2 Fiberglass
dermatitis: tiny papules and
scratch marks

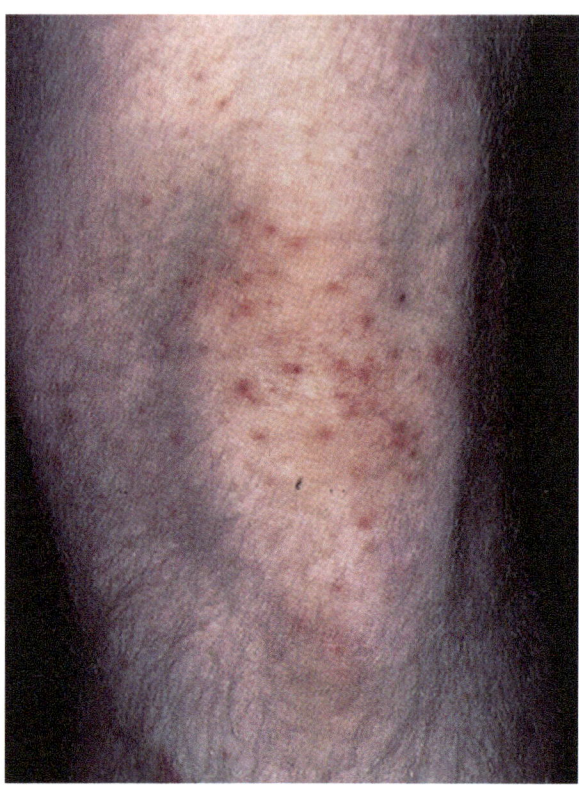

Table 9.2 Clinical signs and symptoms of fiberglass dermatitis

Subjective symptoms	Subjective symptoms are always present. Itching, stinging, and burning sensations are the usual complaints of many patients, with or without objective signs. In particular, facial complaints are not often accompanied by detectable lesions; they correspond to the so-called subjective irritant dermatitis. The eyelids, cheeks, nasal folds, and neck are commonly involved
	Subjective symptoms may occur not only on covered parts of the body, mainly in the flexures (axillae, groins, cubital, and/or popliteal fossae), but also on the extensor aspects of the limbs or on the trunk
Objective symptoms	Objective symptoms are usually present but vary in severity from case to case. Scratch marks, tiny papules, and a maculopapular rash are the usual lesions
	Severe cases could involve secondary infection (pustules) from scratching
	The occurrence of these objective symptoms is highly characteristic and, combined with anamnestic data, usually diagnostic. Nevertheless, when the hands are also involved, differential diagnosis with human scabies has to be kept in mind, and the search for *Sarcoptes scabiei* is advisable

The clinical signs and symptoms of fiberglass dermatitis are described in Table 9.2. They can be extrapolated to other types of fibers.

9.5.2   ABCD due to Dust Particles

Two different situations have to be taken into consideration:

1. The dust particles are "chemically inert." Skin symptoms are related to the mechanical (frictional) properties of particles. It is not clear whether the shape of the particles (e.g., particles with sharp edges) plays an important role or not. Many other concomitant factors are most probably important, such as ambient heat, low humidity, sweating, and/or atopic state. The clinical symptoms are quite similar to those observed with fibers. Facial complaints are usually prominent: the eyelids, cheeks, nasal folds, retroauricular folds, and neck are commonly involved. Workers wearing ill-fitted masks sometimes complain of itching of the face, due to the accumulation of dust under the mask, particularly in the nasal folds. Subjective and objective complaints can also occur on covered parts of the body, due to the accumulation of dust particles under the garments. Indeed, solid particles can pass easily under protective clothes, most often between sleeves and gloves; dust particles can also accumulate on the skin of the feet, even when workers wear safety shoes. Exposure to sawdust is a common problem, encountered worldwide, as emphasized in a recent review article [11].

2. The dust particles are not chemically inert. They release irritant substances (acidic, alkaline, or neutral) that are responsible for true irritant (i.e., chemically induced) contact dermatitis. When dust material is suspended in distilled water, the pH of the supernatant can be very alkaline. Dried industrial dyes show a wide range of pH. In these various situations, clinical symptoms are unequivocally typical of irritant contact dermatitis. Eyelids are preferentially involved, due not only to the accumulation of particles, but also to the increased penetration of chemicals into the skin. Periorbital dermatitis is a common problem encountered in occupational dermatology. Differential diagnosis of this entity is often difficult. Irritant ABCD to dust particles has to be taken into consideration as a potential etiological factor [12].

9.5.3   ABCD due to Sprays, Vapors, and Gases

On the contrary of fibers and/or dust particles dermatitis that may affect covered as well as uncovered parts of the body, occupational irritant ABCD related to sprays, vapors (Fig. 9.3), and/or gases is almost exclusively limited to uncovered parts.

The face and neck are primarily involved. Clinical symptoms are typical of irritant contact dermatitis. Itching, stinging, and burning sensations are the usual complaints. They precede the occurrence of a maculopapular rash. The lesions may be limited to the eyelids (periorbital dermatitis) or extend to the whole face and neck, sparing some partly protected areas, such as retroauricular folds or the margins of the scalp. Organic solvents, ammonia, and formaldehyde are often mentioned as common offending agents, but many others can be listed, such as acids and alkalis, domestic products (e.g., cleansing products), industrial solvents, carbonless copy paper, or phenol vapors.

Fig. 9.3 Irritant ABCD from formaldehyde vapors. The patch test to formaldehyde was negative

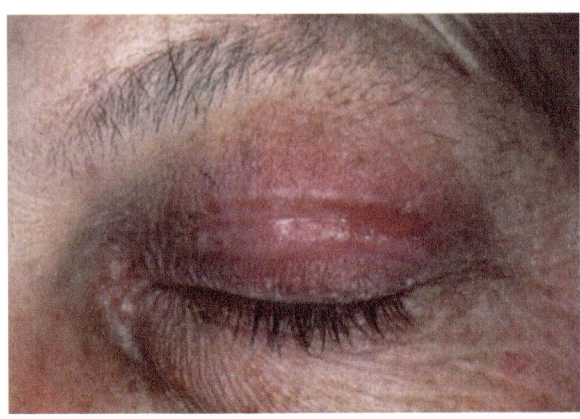

9.5.4 Allergic ABCD

Occupational allergic ABCD is a problem of uppermost importance in our diversified environment, as a result of constant changes in technology.

Airborne "contact" allergens can be volatile (vapors and/or gases), or transported under the form of sprays (mini-droplets), or present in dust particles: all physical forms are common in the work environment.

Clinical symptoms are typical of allergic contact dermatitis (Figs. 9.4 and 9.5). There is no specific sign in relation to airborne contact. Eczematous lesions are symmetrical in most cases; they are acute or chronic, depending on the environmental conditions: nature and/or concentration of the allergens, frequency of airborne contact, and so on. For instance, dermatitis from wood dust normally starts on the eyelids or the lower half of the face, often preceded by a period of itching. Swelling and redness spread to the neck, hands, and forearms. By the time the patient goes for treatment, a diffuse dermatitis, distinctly limited at the margins of the sleeves and collar, might have developed. Because of the accumulation of dust and sweat, the elbow flexures and the skin under a tight collar are often lichenified. Therefore, there is no magic clue that leads to an unequivocal diagnosis. Anamnestic data, analysis of symptoms, and patch test results are needed to reach a correct conclusion.

9.5.5 Phototoxic (Photo Irritant) ABCD and Photoallergic ABCD

Phototoxic and/or photoallergic chemicals can be airborne. Practically, there is no clinical sign that allows a clear-cut distinction between direct contact and airborne contact. Both produce a similar type of eruption. On theoretical grounds, phototoxic reactions are more sharply demarcated, whereas photoallergic reactions display ill-defined margins (Fig. 9.6), but there are many exceptions to the general rule. On the other hand, it can be claimed that in non-airborne phototoxic or photoallergic

Fig. 9.4 Allergic ABCD from cement dust. The potassium dichromate patch test was positive

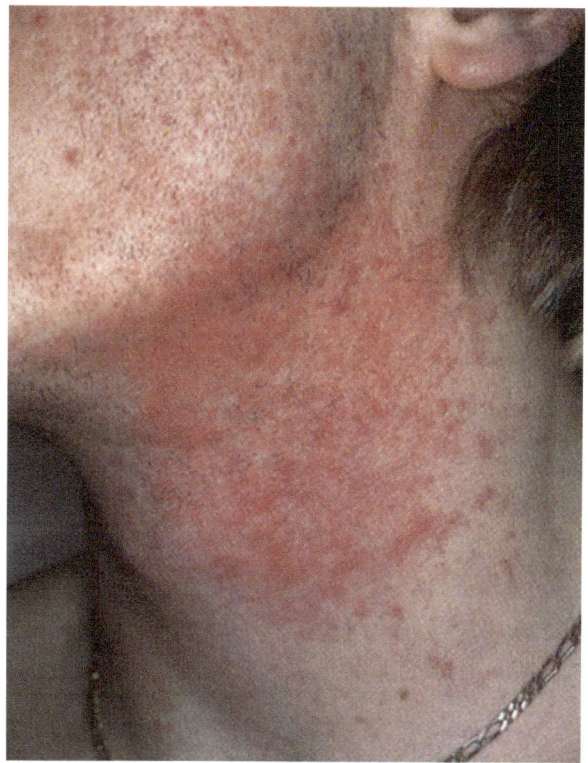

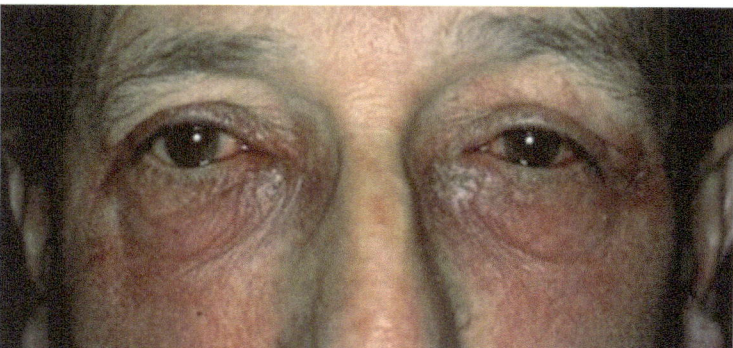

Fig. 9.5   Allergic ABCD from epoxy resin. The patch test to epoxy resin was positive

reactions, some parts of the face are relatively or completely spared, whereas in airborne ones, no part is spared. Once again, the rule has many exceptions. Diagnosis is therefore based on carefully completed anamnestic data, analysis of symptoms and signs, and patch test and photopatch test results [13, 14].

Fig. 9.6 Photoallergic ABCD from powdered pig feed. The patch test and the photopatch test to olaquindox, a piglet feed additive, were positive

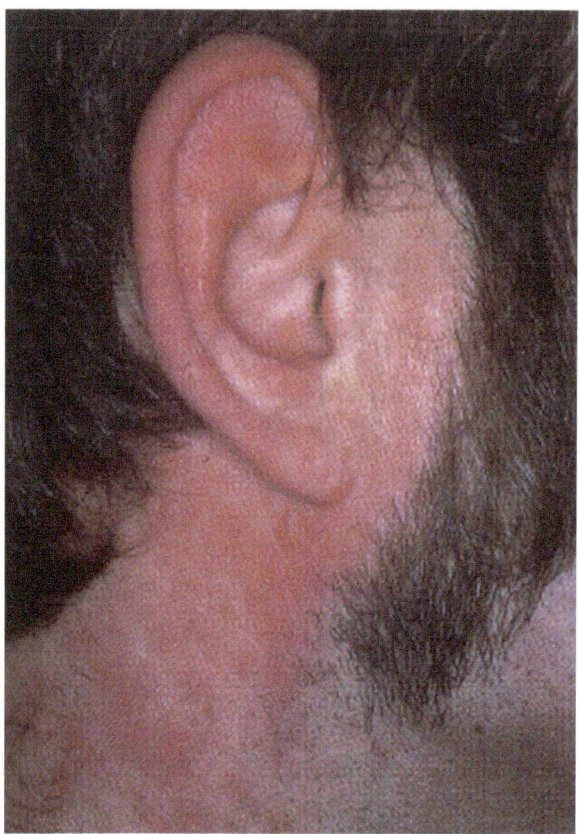

9.5.6 Occupational Airborne (Immunological and Non-immunological) Contact Urticaria

Occupational contact urticaria (either immunological or non-immunological) is well documented in many papers [15]. Due to the abundant literature in the field, it is out of the scope of this chapter, and we refer the reader to general reviews [15].

Airborne contact urticaria to latex proteins is a major problem and is discussed in numerous scientific publications [16, 17].

9.5.7 Exacerbation of "Extrinsic" Atopic Dermatitis by Aeroallergens

It is convincingly proven that patients suffering from atopic dermatitis of exposed sites (the so-called face and neck dermatitis) are made worse by airborne contact with aeroallergens, especially house dust mite [18]. The lesions involve the whole face (including the scalp), the neck, and the décolleté (Fig. 9.7), without any spare

Fig. 9.7 Exacerbation of atopic dermatitis: face and neck dermatitis

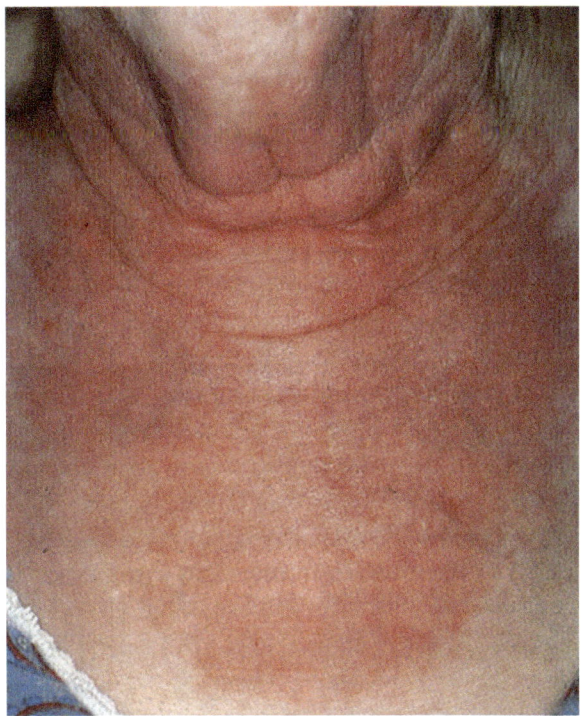

area. They are eczematous, most often dry, scaly, and lichenified. Itching and scratching are very prominent features.

A recent study [19] has shown that 77 % of patients presented with a positive atopy patch test reaction to human dust mite (20 % in pet; Chemotechnique) at day 4, as well as an elevated allergen-specific IgE level. This emphasizes the new concept of "extrinsic" atopic dermatitis, related to filaggrin haploinsufficiency in the stratum corneum; this allows an increased penetration of high-molecular-weight allergens into the skin. The impact of these studies has to be further evaluated in occupational dermatology.

A global evaluation of the sensitivity and the specificity of atopic patch tests has been published recently [20]; it takes into consideration the limitations of the procedure.

9.6 Criteria of Differential Diagnosis Between Allergic ABCD and Photoallergic Contact Dermatitis

This section is considered very important, because it is a good example of the semeiological approach (signs and symptoms) to the differential diagnosis, revisited nowadays in the various fields of dermatology, whereas internal medicine is more and more based upon biological investigations.

Table 9.3 Criteria of differential diagnosis between allergic ABCD and photoallergic contact dermatitis

	Allergic ABCD	Photoallergic contact dermatitis
Clinical signs	Acute dermatitis (most often)	Acute dermatitis
	Affecting the whole face and neck	Affecting the whole face and neck
	Not sparing the so-called shadow areas, i.e., the eyelids (edematous), retroauricular folds, V-shaped area of the anterior aspect of the neck	Sparing to some extent the so-called shadow areas, i.e., the eyelids, retroauricular folds, V-shaped area of the anterior aspect of the neck
Patch testing	Some of the conventional patch tests to suspected allergens are positive	Conventional patch tests are negative
Photopatch testing	Photopatch tests are negative, but some positive patch test reactions can be worsened by UV light (when photopatch-tested)	Some photopatch tests are positive

Criteria of differential diagnosis between allergic ABCD and photoallergic contact dermatitis are presented in Table 9.3.

Nevertheless, it has to be mentioned that these differential characteristics are only indicative; indeed, when phototoxic (photo irritant) and/or photoallergic ABCD is suspected, there is some overlapping of the aforementioned criteria.

9.7 Diagnostic Procedures and Tips Applicable to the Various Classes of ABCD

9.7.1 Preliminary Note

In a recent Danish paper [21], authors developed a tool for systematic "stepwise assessment" of exposures in the work environment, consisting of six steps spanning medical history and workplace visits. All patients referred for a suspicion of occupational contact dermatitis underwent a clinical examination, the stepwise exposure assessment, and extensive patch and prick testing.

This methodology may obviously be applied to ABCD. The order of the steps varies slightly between the departments of occupational dermatology.

9.7.2 Our Multistep Strategy to Reach an Accurate Etiological Diagnosis of ABCD

For many years, we have adopted in our department a multistep strategy [7, 13], which is presented in detail in Table 9.4.

Some additional procedures are available when ABCD to fibers, dust particles, vapors, or gases is suspected (Table 9.5).

Table 9.4 Our multistep strategy to reach an accurate etiological diagnosis of ABCD

1.	At the first visit of the patient at the outpatient clinic, the first, most important step is the precise recording of anamnestic data, clinical symptoms, and exacerbation (or not) at work and determination of the occurrence of all offending agents at the workplace
2.	At the same visit, if allergic and/or photoallergic ABCD is highly suspected, we consider it advisable to first perform a series of patch tests: baseline, oriented additional series related to personal history, i.e., rubber, acrylates, plastic or cosmetic series, etc., and eventually photopatch tests with the standard series of photoallergens. It is a preliminary useful approach to the problem Of course, patch testing with liquid and/or solid products brought by the patient is nonsense, since we ignore their chemical content
3.	The next step is the visit of the dermatologist at the workplace (with the occupational physician) and, concomitantly, taking the necessary steps to obtain from the manufacturer(s) the complete chemical composition of the products
4.	When these investigations have been completed, it is the appropriate time to patch test with the end products, not as such, but following the procedures described in other chapters, concerning extraction of chemicals and the use of semi-open and/or ROATs

Table 9.5 Other specific procedures recommended when irritant ABCD to fibers, dust particles, vapors, or gases is suspected

1.	Collection of samples (i.e., suspected fibers, dust, or liquids sprayed in the air)
2.	Analysis of samples, including pH, physical and chemical properties of chemicals, etc.
3.	Determination of the presence of particles (and eventually of chemicals) in the skin (i.e., using skin surface biopsy)
4.	Evaluation of the irritant potential of collected materials on the skin of workers or volunteers by means of noninvasive techniques (such as transepidermal water loss, erythrometry, laser Doppler flowmetry, and others)
5.	Evaluation of the relative rate of humidity in the air
6.	Use of an exposure chamber designed for experiments with controlled exposure to airborne particles, mainly skin and respiratory allergens and irritants. The aims are to study skin effects and to develop methods for the measurement of the deposition of particles on the skin [22, 30]

9.8   Sick Building Syndrome (SBS)

Sick building syndrome (SBS) is a specific indoor skin condition, characterized by a group of symptoms occurring rather commonly, in particular, among office workers but also in industrial settings. It affects more or less simultaneously a cohort of subjects working together in the same building.

The complaints are heterogeneous, such as irritable dry skin, facial flushing, itching, prickling, tingling or burning sensations, perception of unusual odors, dryness, and cracking of mucous membranes of mouth, nose, and eyes, often associated with recurrent sore throat, headache, fatigue, and loss of concentration.

These subjective symptoms are often disconcerting for the practitioner (dermatologist or occupational physician) because objective signs are either absent or of minor importance.

But the reality of the syndrome is unquestionable, and many papers have been focused on diagnostic procedures in order to solve and to prevent the occurrence of those various symptoms [23–25].

The etiological factors are diversified and often intricate; they are classified in two categories: (1) physicochemical and (2) psychosocial.

Globally, when SBS does occur inside a building or at a workplace, it is of prime importance to appreciate the so-called indoor air quality (IAQ). This is often defined as the extent to which human requirements are met. But what requirements do people have in relation to indoor air? The desire is that the air be perceived as fresh and pleasant, that it has no negative impact on their health, and that the air is stimulating and promotes their work, i.e., that it increases their productivity [26].

The main causes incriminated in the onset of SBS are listed in Table 9.6. This list is intended to be a guide for the physician in charge of the problem.

Apart from correcting all these potential nuisances, a general psychosocial strategy is recommended, and we have applied it systematically in our department [13].

Some courses of action are detailed in Table 9.7.

Table 9.6 Main causes incriminated in the onset of SBS

1.	Inappropriate ventilation related to mechanical ventilation systems and/or internal air conditioning (in case of no regular replacement of filter collecting dust particles) [27]
2.	Insufficient relative humidity delivered in the air. When its rate is under 30 %, SBS can be expected to occur [28]
3.	Tobacco smoking indoors. It is strictly forbidden in many countries but not in all [29]
4.	Indoor air pollution by interior decoration materials has recently become a major health problem. The presence of fibers (fiberglass or others) and/or dust particles cannot be excluded. But, in the majority of cases, volatile chemicals are responsible (i.e., formaldehyde or organic compounds such as butanol or 1,2-dichloroethane). Air is collected using a diffusion sampler and measured by GC/MS [30]. Identifiable aeroallergens such as pollens may also be present in the air
5.	Work stress plays often an important role in the occurrence of SBS. It is manifested by role conflict, work overload, managerial difficulties, and workplace building renovations. All these factors have been significantly associated with perceptions of poor workplace air quality and increased dermatological symptoms of SBS
	In this context, differential diagnosis between SBS and "mass psychogenic illness" has to be taken into consideration

Table 9.7 A psychosocial strategy intended to solve the problems encountered in the SBS syndrome

1.	Limit the number of external consultants to avoid divergent opinions. In case of skin complaints, the advice of only one consultant dermatologist is recommended
2.	Be wary of "negative" attitudes of employers and consultants, who minimize or deny the existence of problems at the risk of aggravating the situation
3.	Do not send the workers to a hospital, to avoid rumor. Call the consultants in the company. They conduct their mission at the workplace and/or in adequate premises
4.	When an epidemic of complaints does occur, gather affected workers in a definite zone, to avoid "psychological contagion"

Table 9.7 (continued)

5. Involve the workers in the search for the causes. Ideally, via the Committee of Safety and Hygiene
6. Communicate in a very open way with the workers, to avoid the dissemination of the rumors
7. Communicate also in a cautious and effective way with the media to avoid the distribution of erroneous information
8. Avoid delivering a premature definitive conclusion on the cause of the problems
9. At the end of the investigations, if no objective cause is revealed (it can be the case in certain epidemics), express the opinion that the problem was connected to stress. Such an explanation is valid only if the persons in charge of the company immediately put into effect practical solutions – that is, elimination of the presumed agents or generators of stress

Practical Tips

- It has to be kept in mind that ABCD presents a kaleidoscope of diseases, including irritant ABCD, allergic ABCD, phototoxic ABCD, photoallergic ABCD, and the exacerbation of atopic dermatitis (face and neck dermatitis).
- Each individual case of ABCD has its own profile, and diagnostic procedures have to be selected accordingly.
- In this respect, an optional "stepwise assessment" of exposures in the work environment has been developed, but its chronological order is subject to modifications. It is a very useful reminder.
- The tools of investigation at our disposal are numerous. They are briefly quoted in this review, and the reader is invited to consult the other chapters to obtain a full explanation about each of them.
- SBS is described in detail. It is a very complex skin condition that requires the expertise of a skilled dermatologist to reach a diagnosis at the proper time. Diagnostic procedures are not only technical, but also psychosocial.

References

1. Lachapelle J-M. Industrial airborne irritant and allergic contact dermatitis. Contact Dermatitis. 1986;14:137–45.
2. Dooms-Goossens A, De Busschere KM, Gevers DM, Dupré KM, Degreef HJ, Loncke JP, et al. Contact dermatitis caused by airborne agents. J Am Acad Dermatol. 1986;15:1–10.
3. Santos R, Goossens A. An update on airborne contact dermatitis 2001–2006. Contact Dermatitis. 2007;57:353–60.
4. Swinnen I, Goossens A. An update on airborne contact dermatitis 2007–2011. Contact Dermatitis. 2013;68:232–8.
5. Lachapelle J-M. Airborne irritant dermatitis. Chapter 8. In: Chew A-L, Maibach HI, editors. Irritant dermatitis. Berlin: Springer; 2006. p. 71–9.
6. Stam-Westerfeld EB, Coenraads PJ, van der Valk PJ, de Jong MC, Fidler V. Rubbing test responses of the skin to man-made mineral fibres of different diameters. Contact Dermatitis. 1994;31:1–4.

7. Lachapelle J-M. Airborne contact dermatitis. Chapter 20. In: Rustemeyer T, Maibach HI, Elsner P, John SM, editors. Textbook of Kanerva's occupational skin diseases. Berlin: Springer; 2011.
8. Cusano F, Mariano M. Fiberglass dermatitis microepidemic in a primary school. Contact Dermatitis. 2007;57:351–2.
9. Bordel-Gomez MT, Miranda-Romero A. Fibreglass dermatitis: a report of 2 cases. Contact Dermatitis. 2008;59:120–2.
10. Hsieh MY, Guo YL, Shiao JS, Sheu HM. Morphology of glass fibers in electronics workers with fiberglass dermatitis – a scanning electron microscopy study. Int J Dermatol. 2001;40:258–61.
11. Chomiczewska-Skora D. Adverse cutaneous reactions induced by exposure to woods. Med Pr. 2013;64:103–18.
12. Feser A, Mahler V. Periorbital dermatitis: causes, differential diagnosis and therapy. J Dtsch Dermatol Ges. 2009;8:159–66.
13. Lachapelle J-M, Frimat P, Tennstedt D, Ducombs G. Précis de Dermatologie Professionnelle et de l'Environnement. Paris: Masson; 1992. p. 107–11.
14. Lachapelle J-M, Goossens A. Photopatch testing. Chapter 5. In: Lachapelle J-M, Maibach HI, editors. Patch testing and prick testing. A practical guide. Official publication of the ICDRG. 3rd ed. Berlin: Springer; 2012. p. 95–101.
15. Basketter D, Lahti A. Immediate contact reactions. Chapter 7. In: Johansen JD, Frosch PJ, Lepoittevin J-P, editors. Contact dermatitis. 5th ed. Berlin: Springer; 2011. p. 137–41.
16. Reunala T, Alenius H, Turjanmaa K, Palosuo T. Latex allergy and skin. Curr Opin Allergy Clin Immunol. 2004;4:397–401.
17. Ownby DR. A history of latex allergy. J Allergy Clin Immunol. 2002;110 suppl 2:S3–14.
18. Samochokhi Z. Hypersensitivity to aeroallergens in adult patients with atopic dermatitis develops due to different immunological mechanisms. Eur J Dermatol. 2007;17:520–4.
19. Hallai N, Gawkrodger DJ. Patch testing to aeroallergens, especially house dust mite, is often positive in atopics with eczema of the face and hands. J Eur Acad Dermatol Venereol. 2009;23:728–9.
20. Nosbaum A, Nicolas J-F. Atopy patch tests. Chapter 9. In: Lachapelle J-M, Maibach HI, editors. Patch testing and prick testing. A practical guide. Official publication of the ICDRG. 3rd ed. Berlin: Springer; 2012. p. 137–44.
21. Friis UF, Menné T, Flyvholm M-A, Bonde JPE, Johansen JD. Occupational allergic contact dermatitis diagnosed by a systematic stepwise exposure assessment of allergens in the work environment. Contact Dermatitis. 2013;69:153–63.
22. Liden C, Lundgren L, Skare L, Liden G, Tornling G, Krantz S. A new whole-body exposure chamber for human skin and lung challenge experiments – the generation of wheat flour aerosols. Ann Occup Hyg. 1998;42:541–7.
23. Wittczak T, Walusiak J. "Sick building syndrome": a problem of occupational medicine. Med Pr. 2001;52:369–73.
24. Worgocki PM, Sindell J, Bischoff W, Brundrett G, Fanger PO, Gyntelberg F, et al. Sick building syndrome: a review of 105 papers. Indoor Air. 2002;12:113–28.
25. Marmot AF, Ely J, Stafford M, Stansfeld SA, Warwick E, Marmot MG. Building health: an epidemiological study of "sick building syndrome". Occup Environ Med. 2006;63:282–9.
26. Ole Fanger P. What is IAQ? Indoor Air. 2006;16:328–34.
27. Seppanen O, Fisk WJ. Association of ventilation system type with SBS symptoms in the office worker. Indoor Air. 2002;12:98–112.
28. Engvall K, Norrby C, Norback D. Sick building syndrome in relation to building dampness. Int Arch Occup Environ Health. 2001;74:270–8.
29. Abdel-Hamid MA, A Hakim S, Elokda EE, Mostafa NS. Prevalence and risk factors of sick building syndrome among office workers. J Egypt Public Health Assoc. 2013;88:109–14.
30. Guo P, Yokoyama K, Piao F, Sakai K, Khalequzzaman M, Kamijima M, et al. Sick building syndrome by indoor air pollution in Dalian, China. Int J Environ Res Public Health. 2013;10:1489–504.

Proxy Contact Dermatitis, or Contact Dermatitis "by Proxy" (Consort or Connubial Dermatitis)

10

John McFadden

Contact dermatitis "by proxy" (consort/connubial dermatitis) occurs when exposure to an agent originating from another individual leads to (usually allergic) contact dermatitis. The means of exposure can be through direct contact with another individual [1], airborne [2], or contaminated clothing or bedding [3, 4]. Occasionally, contact dermatitis "by proxy" has an occupational [4] or recreational [5] source.

It may be morphologically typical for allergic contact dermatitis [6]. Alternatively, there may be an unusual morphology such as pseudolymphomatoid appearance [7, 8], nummular eczema [9], or plaque dermatitis [10]. The distribution of the rash can be highly atypical and can be generalized [11], exposed site [10], or unilateral due to only one side being exposed [1, 12]. The pattern can be of a hand corresponding to the dimensions of the individual transferring the suspect agent [13, 14].

Genital exposure can produce a balanitis [15, 16] or a vulvitis [17], which can then develop secondary spread [17].

As contact dermatitis "by proxy" involves exposure to the causative agent through transfer through another individual, the dose will generally be lower than cases through direct contact with the causative agent. Therefore, it is perhaps not surprising that the patients presenting with contact dermatitis "by proxy" usually have a high sensitivity to the causative agent as demonstrated by usually having vigorous patch test reactions, in some cases even being +++ [5, 6, 11, 13, 14, 18].

The demonstration of contact dermatitis from exposure to dyed hair [9, 19] and clothes contaminated from epoxy resin [4] reveals the presence of unpolymerized and uncured products even after the dyeing/curing processes have occurred.

Contact dermatitis "by proxy" is usually not an easy diagnosis to make. It often requires highly skillful history taking, a high index of suspicion, and appropriate

J. McFadden, BM, DM
Department of Cutaneous Allergy, St. John's Institute of Dermatology,
King's College, St. Thomas' Hospital, Lambeth Palace Rd.,
London, SE1 7EH, UK
e-mail: john.mcfadden@kcl.ac.uk

J.-M. Lachapelle et al. (eds.), *Patch Testing Tips*,
DOI 10.1007/978-3-642-45395-3_10, © Springer-Verlag Berlin Heidelberg 2014

patch testing. Consequently, contact dermatitis "by proxy" is probably underdiagnosed. A differential diagnosis of contact dermatitis "by proxy" should be particularly entertained if:

1. There are no obvious direct triggers for the dermatitis from direct contact to allergens/irritants, but the dermatitis does not appear to be endogenous in nature
2. There is no obvious direct exposure to a positive patch test agent
3. The presenting dermatitis has an unusual pattern of distribution or asymmetry
4. There is a bizarre pattern (such as the shape of a hand)
5. Genital dermatitis is present
6. There is an unexplained vigorous positive patch test

10.1 Case Reports

10.1.1 Perfumes and Fragrances

A 25-year-old mechanic presented with large edematous vesicular plaques involving the right cheek, right side of his nose, and left lower eyelid [10]. Patch testing revealed a ++ reaction to the fragrance chemicals *Myroxylon pereirae* and cinnamic alcohol. Further patch testing with his aftershave was also positive. He presented a year later with a striking unilateral facial eczematous eruption on the exposed areas of his face. Although he had carefully avoided fragrances since being diagnosed with allergy, it transpired that two nights before the onset of this latest dermatitis, his wife had applied a fragrance to herself in preparation for a party.

A 40-year-old woman presented with dermatitis on the lateral aspects of the left forearm and upper arm [1]. She was patch test + to *Myroxylon pereirae* and to fragrance mix I. The patient stopped using fragranced products, but it transpired that the husband slept on the left side of the bed and used a variety of fragranced products in large doses. Subsequent patch testing of the patient to the husband's deodorant sprays was positive. There was complete symptomatic relief on discontinuation of fragranced products by her husband.

A 76-year-old woman presented with a 3-month history of a pruritic erythematous rash distributed on the upper part of her chest and neck and her arms [11]. She had no history of dermatitis and denied use of perfumes or cosmetics. Patch testing to a standard and fragrance tray of allergens revealed a +++ reaction to both fragrance mix I and to *Evernia prunastri* (oak moss), a constituent of fragrance mix I. It transpired that her husband regularly used an aftershave containing *Evernia prunastri* at a concentration of 3 %. Patch testing to the aftershave revealed a +++ reaction. When the husband stopped using the aftershave, the dermatitis resolved and did not reappear.

A 69-year-old man presented with a history of intermittent eczema for 20 years [20]. Over the last 2 years it had been persistent. It frequently started on the exposed surfaces of the arms and spread to the neck, trunks, and legs; the face was only occasionally involved. The eczema had been difficult to control and had required both injection of corticosteroids and hospitalization. Patch testing showed a positive reaction to the synthetic fragrance chemical hydroxycitronellal. It transpired that the patient's wife had been a long-term employee of a cosmetics firm and that the husband regularly used his wife's bubble bath and that the wife used their spray perfumes and colognes as air freshener and wore the firm's fragrances. The manufacturer confirmed the presence of hydroxycitronellal in all these products. When the husband stopped using her wife's bubble bath and his wife stopped using the colognes and spray perfume, his condition improved.

10.1.2 Cosmetic Preservative

A 29-year-old woman complained of recurrent vesiculopapular lesions on the limbs [13]. In particular, she had a clear hand-form lesion on her right thigh after the recent use of a moisturizing hand cream used by her husband. She gave a history of reacting to different cosmetics over a long period of time. Application of the suspected cream on the antecubital area resulted in an eczematous lesion developing after the first application. There was a +++ reaction on patch testing to methyldibromoglutaronitrile, which was present in her husband's hand cream.

10.1.3 Hair Dye

Mitchell [9] first described a case of contact dermatitis "by proxy" from recently dyed hair. A 25-year-old man presented with nummular eczematous patches on the trunk and upper limbs most concentrated on the upper inner arms and breast. A consensus was reached that the eruption was typical of nummular eczema, with an odd distribution. Patch test was positive to PPD (++), p-aminobenzene (++), and to p-toluenediamine (++). Enquiries revealed that the patient's wife regularly dyed her hair black, and she was accustomed to read a book in bed with her hair "nestled" to his armpit. Patch testing to the wife's hair "as is" also showed a positive reaction (++). Cronin [19] reported a 24-year-old man presenting with a 10-month history of red, weeping patches of eczema on the extensor surfaces of both arms. Patch testing showed a ++ reaction to the wife's hair, +– to para-toluenediamine, and +– to ortho-nitro-para-phenylenediamine. His wife had dyed her hair for 3 years and rested her head on his arms corresponding to the eczematous areas. Warin [12] reports a 39-year-old man presenting with a 2-month history of a recurrent dermatitis affecting the left arm. He had noticed that each time his rash flared up, his partner had dyed her hair black. When seen he had a weeping annular eczema on the left arm. Patch testing showed a ++ to PPD and to the hair dye his wife used. Hindson [21] reported a 21-year-old female dental hygienist presenting with an area of dermatitis on the inner aspect of the left forearm. When working she wore a short-sleeved dress, stood behind her patient, and held her instruments in the right hand and her mirror in the left hand so that her left forearm came into frequent contact with her patient's hair. Patch testing with a baseline series was negative including to PPD, at 48 and 96 h. However, a patch test to ortho-nitro-para-phenylenediamine was strongly positive at 48 h. A diagnosis of proxy contact dermatitis from exposure to her dental patients' dyed hair was made.

A 37-year-old man presented with a 3-month history of an itchy facial rash that later became more generalized over the trunk and upper limbs [7]. He had widespread erythematous tumid plaques. A biopsy showed spongiotic dermatitis with secondary impetiginization. The dermatitis cleared with potent topical steroids. Patch test to standard and cosmetic series showed a ++ positive reaction to PPD. It transpired that his partner regularly dyed her hair, and applications were associated with flares in his rash. He presented 6 months later with the same tumid plaques, despite his wife using a new hair dye, and histology this time showed a lymphomatoid dermatitis picture. The new hair dye contained the aromatic amine toluene-2,5-diamine sulfate, which is known to be able to cross-react with PPD. On discontinuing this product, his rash cleared up. A similar case was that of a 32-year-old man with infiltrated lesions on the left arm with eczematous lesions of the waist [8]. Biopsy showed a dense lymphoid infiltrate. A PPD patch test was the only positive result on screening with a baseline series. The only source of exposure to PPD found was the use of hair dye by the spouse, and withdrawal of the allergen resulted in complete remission.

The concept of proxy dermatitis from exposure to recently dyed hair is in keeping with a recent report that substantive amounts of unconsumed precursors and couplers are present on hair after the dyeing process [22].

10.1.4 Plant Products in Cosmetics

A 25-year-old metal worker presented with recurrent facial dermatitis on the eyelids, cheeks, and perioral area [6]. The rash worsened on Mondays. He was found to be patch test + to sesquiterpene lactones (SL) mix 0.1 % pet. Further investigation led to him being patch tested to his girlfriend's cosmetics. Reading at day 4 showed +++ reaction to a makeup (containing *Matricaria parthenium*) and a deodorant (containing *Laurus nobilis* and *Anthemis nobilis*). The patient was diagnosed as having allergic contact dermatitis due to SLs in his girlfriend's products.

10.1.5 Medicament Sources

Baeck and Goossens [2] reviewed patch test results and sensitization sources in patients who reacted positively to corticosteroids tested in the Leuven Dermatology Department over an 18-year period. They found 15 subjects, not themselves treated by budesonide-containing aerosols, but taking care of/or living together with patients who used them, appeared to have been sensitized by airborne exposure and/or airborne allergic contact dermatitis. The nine patients presenting with suspected airborne contact dermatitis to the budesonide presented with eyelid and/or facial eczema. Another individual presented with a 3-month history of recurrent vesiculobullous lesions on the dorsum of the right hand, sometimes extending to the forearm and arm [18]. Patch testing revealed a positive reaction to budesonide 0.01 % pet. (++). It transpired that he had contact with budesonide spray during asthma treatment for his 2-year-old daughter. The patient began avoiding exposure to the budesonide-containing aerosol, and no more episodes of dermatitis have occurred since.

A 30-year-old physician presented with a pruritic eruption well localized to the right side of the neck and right anterior axillary fold [3]. Although he had not been using topical preparations, he had mentioned that he had given his wife 5 % benzoyl peroxide for mild acne on the back. Patch testing was strongly positive to benzoyl peroxide. The authors assume that, as the patient lay on the left side of the bed, the right side of his neck/axilla would be in contact with bedsheets that could have been contaminated with benzoyl peroxide. Since the wife discontinued use of the preparation, there were no further problems.

A 22-year-old woman had labial urticaria with oropharyngeal edema several minutes after kissing her boyfriend, who had taken amoxicillin a few minutes beforehand [23]. Previously she had suffered from generalized urticaria after she had taken amoxicillin. A prick test with amoxicillin was positive, and a diagnosis of consort contact urticaria was made.

10.1.6 Genital Contact

Hindson [24] reported on allergic contact dermatitis to rubber accelerators in condoms over a 10-year period at St. John's Institute, London. Although the great majority of patients presenting were males ($n=33$), there were also two females who presented with pruritus vulvae.

A 40-year-old man developed acute pruritic erythema, erosions, and edema of the glans penis and prepuce less than 24 h after intercourse. Slight balanitis had been noticed 3 months previously. On questioning it was found that his wife had used a lubricating gel containing chlorhexidine 0.03 %. Patch testing with chlorhexidine gluconate 0.5 % aq. and the lubricating gel was ++ for both at day 2 and 3.

A 44-year-old man presented with recurrent balanitis [15]. His wife had been using a localized spermicide containing phenylmercuric nitrate. Patch testing to mercury was positive.

A 35-year-old man presented with acute vesicular dermatitis, especially on the glans penis but spreading to the abdomen and upper thighs. His wife's vulvovaginitis had been treated with pessaries containing clotrimazole. He was patch test positive to clotrimazole 1 % eth. The dermatitis cleared after discontinuation of treatment.

Kint et al. [25] report a young atopic woman presenting with burning of the vulva and vulvovaginal area during or after coitus, followed by vesiculation, lichenification, and the development of generalized eczema. She was found on investigation to have a type I and possible type IV allergy to human seminal plasma, as well as type I allergy to latex.

10.1.7 Occupational Sources

A 10-year-old girl presented with a dermatitis on the right side of her abdomen forming the shape of a hand, identical in dimensions to her mother's [14]. The mother was a hairdresser and handled various cosmetic and hair products. Patch testing showed positive reactions to benzothiazole (+++), methyldibromoglutaronitrile (++), and essential oils (++), and a diagnosis of consort allergic contact dermatitis was made. The mother was then instructed regarding prevention of her daughter's contact to these agents by contamination of the mother's hands.

A 54-year-old woman presented with a 4-day history of dermatitis of her neck and face, particularly the eyelids. Two years previously she had presented with a similar rash and, among other agents, was found on patch testing to be allergic to epoxy resin (++). Twenty-four hours before the current episode, she had visited her son, who worked in a factory preparing epoxy paints. As his washing machine was not working, she had hand washed his work-soiled clothes. A diagnosis of epoxy-by-proxy dermatitis was made.

10.1.8 From Recreational Activity (Dancing)

A 40-year-old woman presented with a figurate, acute eczematous reaction involving her right hand, back waist, and left foot. She had been giving tango lessons in the evening and suspected that the dermatitis was related to close body contact while dancing [5]. One of her students admitted using ketoprofen topical medications. The patient reacted strongly to ketoprofen (+++ photoaggravated) and was deemed to be responsible for past sensitization from personal use and for the current photoexacerbated allergic contact dermatitis triggered by consort contact. Schmutz and Trechot [26] also report a case of consort allergic contact dermatitis from ballroom dancing.

10.1.9 Photodermatitis

Wilkinson [27] described two cases. The first was a 67-year-old man who presented with a severe photodermatitis that persisted through summer. He denied taking any drugs, and the rash persisted when all possible contact causes were removed. It was only then that he mentioned that over this period of time his wife had been unable to swallow her chlorpromazine tablets and that he had been in the habit of crushing these on the kitchen table. When her medication was changed, his rash cleared up and did not recur.

The second case was of a 35-year-old wife of a veterinary surgeon who developed a severe photodermatitis. She was not using photosensitizing drugs nor using any known photosensitizing topical agents. She did occasionally drive her husband's car, in which he carried drugs including chlorpromazine and phenothiazine. She was photopatch test positive to chlorpromazine and phenothiazine. The patient confirmed that there was always a certain amount of dust in the car from spillage or breakage of the drugs in traveling over farm roads. A change of car and more stringent control of packing of the drugs were accompanied by a gradual resolution of the dermatitis.

Practical Tips

- Contact dermatitis "by proxy" (consort/connubial dermatitis) represents a contact dermatitis (usually allergic) to an agent originating from another individual.
- Agents involved include fragrances, hair dyes, other cosmetic agents, medicaments, and chemicals applied to the genitalia.
- Exposure to the offending agent can be through direct contact with the other individual, airborne, or from contaminated clothing or bedding. Occasionally, sources of exposure can be from a recreational or occupational source.
- Patterns of dermatitis can be very atypical and often asymmetrical. Unless suspected the history can be of the dermatitis appearing at irregular and seemingly unexplained intervals.
- The morphology can be either classical or atypical.
- Affected individuals are often highly sensitive to the allergic agent.
- Diagnosis of contact dermatitis "by proxy" can only be achieved through skillful history taking, a high index of suspicion, and appropriate patch testing.

References

1. Jensen P, Ortiz PG, Hartmann-Petersen S, Sandby-Moller J, Menné T, Thyssen JP, et al. Connubial allergic contact dermatitis caused by fragrance ingredients. Dermatitis. 2012;23(1): e1–2.
2. Baeck M, Goossens A. Patients with airborne sensitization/contact dermatitis from budesonide-containing aerosols 'by proxy'. Contact Dermatitis. 2009;61:1–8.
3. Caro I. Connubial contact dermatitis to benzoyl peroxide. Contact Dermatitis. 1976;2(6):362.
4. Lyon CC, Beck MH. Epoxy-by-proxy dermatitis. Contact Dermatitis. 2000;42:306.
5. Gallo R, Paolino S, Marcella G, Parodi A. Consort allergic contact dermatitis caused by ketoprofen in a tango dancer. Contact Dermatitis. 2010;63:172–4.
6. Bernedo N, Audicana MT, Uriel O, Velasco M, Gastaminza G, Fernández E, et al. Allergic contact dermatitis from cosmetics applied by the patient's girlfriend. Contact Dermatitis. 2004;50:252–3.
7. Veysey EC, Burge S, Cooper S. Consort contact dermatitis to paraphenylenediamine, with an unusual clinical presentation of tumid plaques. Contact Dermatitis. 2007;56:366–7.
8. Hospital V, Amarger S, Franck F, Ferrier Le Bouëdec MC, Souteyrand P, D'Incan M, et al. Proxy lymphomatoid contact dermatitis. Ann Dermatol Venereol. 2011;138(4):315–8.
9. Mitchell JC. Allergic dermatitis from paraphenylenediamine presenting as nummular eczema. Contact Dermatitis Newsl. 1972;11:270.
10. Swinter LJ. Connubial dermatitis from perfumes. Contact Dermatitis. 1980;6:226.

11. Held JL, Rusakowski AM, Deleo VA. Consort contact dermatitis due to oak moss. Arch Dermatol. 1988;124:261–2.
12. Warin AP. Contact dermatitis to partner's hair dye. Clin Exp Dermatol. 1976;1:283–4.
13. Lujan-Rodriguez D, Penate-Santana Y, Hernandez-Machin B, Borrego L. Connubial allergic contact dermatitis to Euxyl K 400. Contact Dermatitis. 2006;54:122–3.
14. Sfia M, Dhaoui MA, Doss N. Consort allergic dermatitis to cosmetic agents in a 10-year old girl. Contact Dermatitis. 2007;57:56–7.
15. Bonnetblanc JM, Delrous JL. Connubial dermatitis from phenylmercuric nitrate. Contact Dermatitis. 1996;34:367.
16. Barazza V. Connubial allergic contact balanitis due to chlorhexidine. Contact Dermatitis. 2001;45:42.
17. Valsecchi R, Pansera B, de Landro A, Cainelli T. Connubial contact sensitization to clotrimazole. Contact Dermatitis. 1994;30:248.
18. Teixeira V, Coutinho I, Goncalo M. Budesonide allergic contact dermatitis "by proxy"? Dermatitis. 2013;24:144–6.
19. Cronin E. Dermatitis from wife's dyed hair. Contact Dermatitis Newsl. 1973;13:363.
20. Mathias T, Cram D, Ragsdale J, Maibach HI. Contact dermatitis caused by spouse's perfume and cologne. Can Med Assoc J. 1978;119:257–8.
21. Hindson C. O-Nitro paraphenylenediamine in hair dye- an unusual dental hazard. Contact Dermatitis. 1975;1:333.
22. Rastogi SC, Sosted H, Johansen J, Menné T, Bossi R. Unconsumed precursors and couplers after formation of oxidative hair dyes. Contact Dermatitis. 2006;55(2):95–100.
23. Petavy-Catala C, Machet L, Vaillant L. Consort contact urticaria due to amoxicillin. Contact Dermatitis. 2011;44:251.
24. Hindson TC. Studies I contact dermatitis. xvi contraceptives. Trans St John's Hosp Dermatol Soc. 1966;52:1–4.
25. Kint B, Degreef H, Dooms-Goossens A. Combined allergy to human seminal plasma and latex: case report and review of the literature. Contact Dermatitis. 1994;30(1):7–11.
26. Schmutz JL, Trechot P. Ballroom dancing and consort allergic contact dermatitis. Ann Dermatol Venereol. 2011;138(11):803–4.
27. Wilkinson DS. Connubial photodermatitis. Contact Dermatitis. 1975;1:58.

Semi-open (or Semi-occlusive) Tests

11

An E. Goossens

Patch testing remains, at present, the golden standard to identify a contact allergen, and it should be performed as extensively as possible in order to cover all potential allergens a particular subject is in contact with. Besides patch testing, other types of skin tests, such as open and semi-open tests, repeated open application tests (ROAT), usage tests, and even prick tests (in order to diagnose contact urticaria and/or protein contact dermatitis), may need to be performed. We will focus here on semi-open (or semiocclusive) tests, which are useful modifications for products that have a certain irritation potential [1–4].

11.1 Method

The *semi-open test* consists of direct application, with a cotton Q-tip, of a minute amount (1–2 µL) of a liquid on a skin surface of about 1 cm^2 (Figs. 11.1 and 11.2). After complete evaporation of the liquid (the excess can be removed with a paper filter or another Q-tip), the *completely dry* test site is then covered with acrylic tape (Fig. 11.3). Diluted products (e.g., 1–2 % aqueous) also can be tested this way. The reading of the skin test is performed as with regular patch testing (Figs. 11.4 and 11.5).

11.2 Purpose

- Have access to a practical and rapid method in case multiple products need to be tested.
- Avoid false-positive or irritant reactions by patch testing potentially irritating products; this does not mean that a semi-open test cannot give rise to an irritant

A.E. Goossens, RPharm, PhD
Department of Dermatology, Katholieke Universiteit Leuven,
Kapucijnenvoer 33, Leuven 3000, Belgium
e-mail: an.goossens@uzleuven.be

J.-M. Lachapelle et al. (eds.), *Patch Testing Tips*,
DOI 10.1007/978-3-642-45395-3_11, © Springer-Verlag Berlin Heidelberg 2014

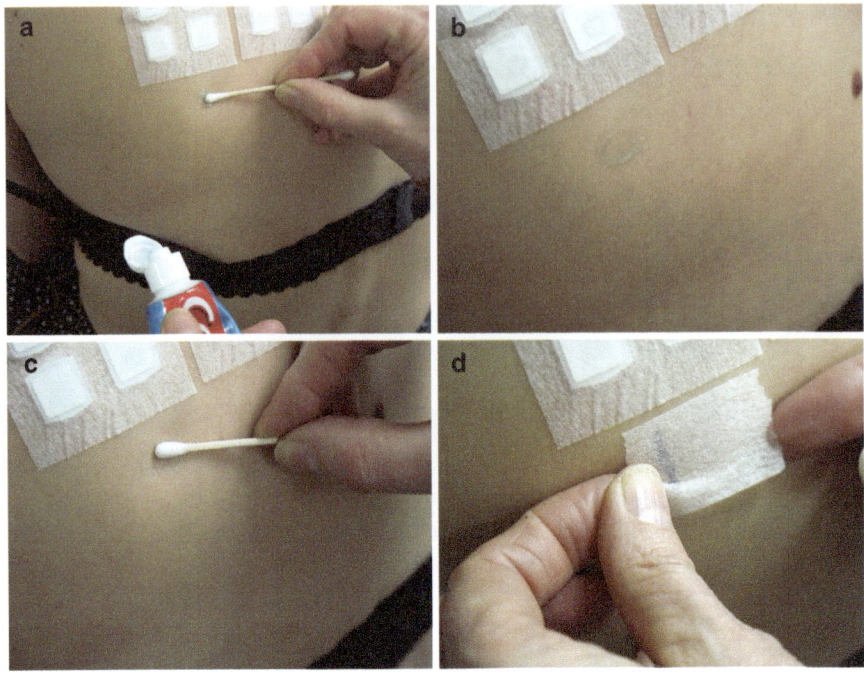

Fig. 11.1 Semi-open test: method of application

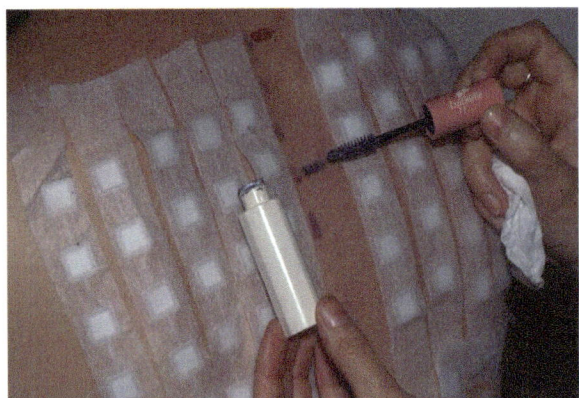

Fig. 11.2 Semi-open test with mascara

Fig. 11.3 Strong positive semi-open test to a shampoo. The patient was allergic to cocamidopropyl betaine present in it

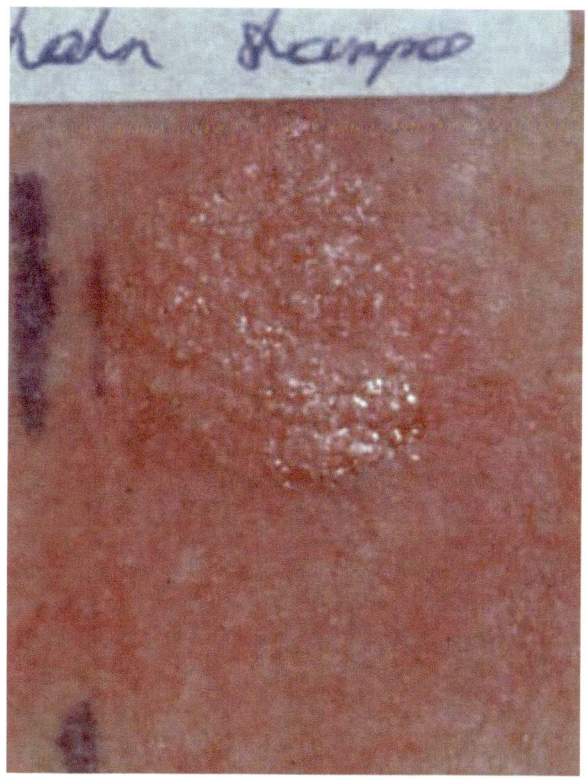

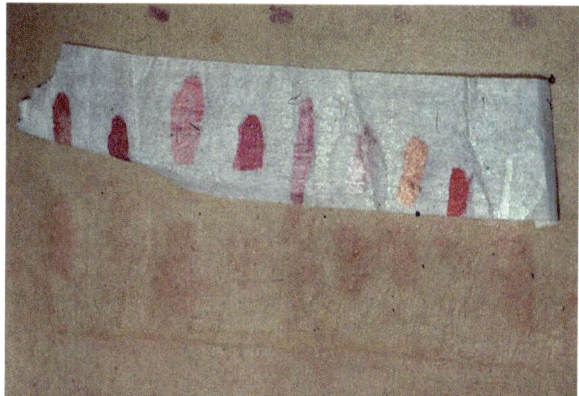

Fig. 11.4 Result of semi-open tests with nail varnish

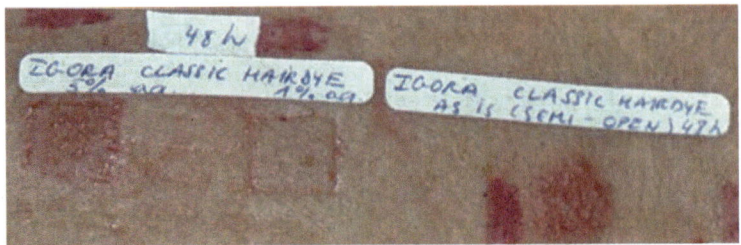

Fig. 11.5 Comparison of positive reactions obtained with a semi-open test and a 1 and 2 % dilution of a hair dye

response. This explains why some basic knowledge about the nature of the product is absolutely necessary.

- Avoid false-negative reactions by testing products that are too diluted – for example, in case of a contact allergy to a fragrance ingredient, a hair dye (see Fig. 11.5), or a preservative in a shampoo. However, in case of a negative semi-open test, the existence of a contact allergy might not be discarded either: it is indeed possible that the allergen is present in a concentration too low to produce a positive test. This also points to the importance of testing with all ingredients separately, in an appropriate concentration and vehicle, in case a contact allergy is really suspected.

11.3   Conditions of Use

This test method is not based on scientific research but on a long-standing expertise.

The performance of the semi-open test depends mainly on the nature of the products the patient brings with him/her. The actual-use conditions and the way in which the product is in contact with the skin need to be taken into account. The golden rule is that when direct skin contact or contamination may occur while handling the product, either on purpose (e.g., shampoos and soaps or other cleaning products) or accidentally (e.g., paints, soluble oils), then the product may be tested in this way. Corrosive or other toxic materials (pH < 3 or >10) that are normally used in closed systems only or with appropriate protective clothing or completely unknown products are completely excluded from testing! Moreover, highly acidic or alkaline products are not tested unless they are buffered [5].

Hence, numerous products with a (slight) irritant potential can be tested using the semi-open test method, provided that the results are interpreted carefully and confirmed by testing with diluted products and certainly with the individual ingredients. Examples include topical pharmaceutical products such as antiseptic agents, products containing solvents such as propylene glycol in high concentrations, and creams based on the emulsifier sodium lauryl sulfate; cosmetic products containing emulsifiers, solvents, or other substances with an irritant potential, such as mascara, nail lacquers, hair dyes, shampoos, permanent-wave solutions, liquid soaps, and peelings; and household and industrial products. After having verified whether the pH is not too low or too high or that a corrosive material is not involved, the semi-open test can be useful for a number of products: paints, resins, varnish, glue, ink, wax, soluble oils, etc.

Practical Tips
- Use semi-open (or semiocclusive) testing for identifying potential aller-genic products that have a certain irritation potential.
- Follow the golden rule: only apply this method when direct skin contact or contamination may occur while handling the product.
- Interpret the results carefully and confirm by testing with diluted products and certainly with the individual ingredients.
- Check the pH of the products.
- Never test corrosive materials.

References

1. Goossens A. Minimizing the risks of missing a contact allergy. Dermatology. 2001;202: 186–9.
2. Lachapelle J-M, Maibach HI. Patch testing and prick testing. a practical guide. 3rd ed. Berlin/Heidelberg: Springer; 2012. p. 114–6.
3. Goossens A. Alternatives aux patch-tests. Ann Dermatol Vénéréol. 2009;136:623–5.
4. Frosch PJ, Geier J, Uter W, Goossens A. Patch testing with the patient's own materials. Chapter 57. In: Contact dermatitis. 5th ed. Berlin/Heidelberg: Springer; 2011. p. 1107–19.
5. Bruze M. Use of buffer solutions for patch testing. Contact Dermatitis. 1984;10:267–9.

The Use of Ultrasonic Bath Extracts in the Diagnostics of Contact Allergy and Allergic Contact Dermatitis

12

Magnus Bruze

12.1 Introduction

To arrive at a diagnosis of allergic contact dermatitis is a three-step procedure in which the first step is establishing the presence of a contact allergy [1]. Thereafter, it shall be demonstrated that there is a present exposure to the sensitizer or possibly cross-reacting substances. Finally, the clinical relevance of the exposure shall be assessed (i.e., does the type and magnitude of the exposure on the one hand and degree of reactivity to the sensitizer on the other explain the dermatitis under investigation with regard to its type, localization, and course). Obviously, the first step, establishing the presence of a contact allergy, is crucial for a diagnosis of allergic contact dermatitis. Without contact allergy, exposure to a hazardous factor may not justify a diagnosis of allergic contact dermatitis but possibly a diagnosis of irritant contact dermatitis [2].

12.2 Establishing a Contact Allergy

Although more than 100 years have passed since the first patch test was performed [3], we still have to rely on this methodology, which repeatedly has been improved over the decades. Indeed, there are in vitro methods available, including lymphocyte transformation test and measurement of cytokine release with ELISA technique, to establish contact allergy [4]. However, these methods exist mainly only for polar substances such as metal salts. They are, therefore, of limited value in daily practice, where contact allergy to various types of chemicals and products needs to be confirmed or ruled out.

M. Bruze, MD, PhD
Department of Occupational and Environmental Dermatology,
Lund University, Jan Waldenströms gata 16, Malmö S-205 02, Sweden
e-mail: magnus.bruze@med.lu.se

J.-M. Lachapelle et al. (eds.), *Patch Testing Tips*,
DOI 10.1007/978-3-642-45395-3_12, © Springer-Verlag Berlin Heidelberg 2014

12.3   Patch Testing

Most patients with a suspected allergic contact dermatitis are patch tested with a base-line series, which usually consists of 25–30 test preparations. These preparations represent chemically defined substances such as nickel and paraphenylenediamine, compound chemicals such as p-tert-butylphenol-formaldehyde resin, and colophony, consisting of many substances, many of which may be unknown, and mixes such as fragrance mix I and thiuram mix. Depending on the history, localization of the dermatitis, and occupation, additional test series representing sensitizers in various occupations and products may be tested. Frequently also patient-supplied products will be tested.

It is important to remember that patch testing is an assay for establishing contact allergy rather than an assay for diagnosis of allergic contact dermatitis, although establishing the presence of contact allergy is the first step in the diagnosis of allergic contact dermatitis. The patch test concentration, or actually more correctly the dose of the sensitizer/cm^2, should be as high as possible to trace any existing contact allergy with due considerations to avoid adverse reactions, particularly active sensitization [5]. Thus, the test concentrations/doses are not and should not reflect the concentrations present in daily-life products such as cosmetics. Usually, the concentrations are 5–20 times higher in the test preparations than in these products [6].

12.4   Patient-Supplied Products

For a more complete investigation on whether a patient suffers from an allergic contact dermatitis, one should also test patient-supplied products representing the occupational and non-occupational environment. Many items and materials such as rubber, textile, paper, and moisturizers can be tested as is, whereas others, such as shampoos, metal-working fluids, glues, and paints, need to be diluted before testing. In case there is a strong suspicion that a product is the culprit of the contact dermatitis, many dermatologists will simultaneously test known contact sensitizers in these products according to the information available from sources such as labeling, the Web, and material safety data sheets. In this way the sensitizers in the products will be patch tested at concentrations 5–20 times higher than in the products [6]. Hereby, the risk of getting a false-negative patch test reaction diminishes. However, what is to be done when a product tested is strongly suspected to be the culprit of the dermatitis but there is no information on separate constituents why testing of ingredients at higher concentrations than present in the product is impossible? When facing this question in the late 1980s, I got the idea to test with ultrasonic bath extracts [7].

12.5   Rationale Behind Patch Testing with Ultrasonic
Bath Extracts

Patch testing with extracts of patient-supplied materials is no novelty. However, usually this extraction procedure has been performed in a non-standardized and time-consuming way. The extraction procedure using an ultrasonic bath means an improved device to get standardized extracts from the same kind of products in a short time with regard to extraction area and time, volume of extracting solvent, use of ultrasonic bath, and evaporation. The idea behind patch testing with ultrasonic bath extracts is to test a possible but unknown contact sensitizer at a higher concentration than what is present in the product, which has yielded a negative reaction when tested as is. For example, if a piece of a rubber item measuring 50 cm^2 is used for extraction and then tested in a small Finn chamber measuring 8 mm in diameter, then there is a possible increase of dose around 100 times (50 cm^2 concentrated into 0.5 cm^2 for a Finn chamber). A large volume of solvent can be used (e.g., 5–20 mL) for extraction and then followed by evaporation of the solvent to dryness. Thereafter, the same or another solvent is added to give a volume of 1 mL of which a small volume (15 µL for a Finn chamber with a diameter of 0.8 cm) can be used for patch testing.

12.6   Indications for the Use of Ultrasonic Bath Extracts

In the diagnostics of allergic contact dermatitis, ultrasonic bath extracts can be used for the two first steps (i.e., establishment of contact allergy and demonstration of exposure to the sensitizer). The major indications for the use of ultrasonic bath extracts are listed in Table 12.1. The first five indications in the table concern establishment of contact dermatitis and the last one, demonstration of exposure to the sensitizer.

12.6.1 Establishing Contact Allergy

The use of ultrasonic bath extracts is a simple method to obtain solutions for patch testing. At our department patients with suspected allergic contact dermatitis are tested at the first visit for reasons of economy and patient convenience. Besides patch testing with our baseline series and possibly additional series, patient-supplied products will be tested at the same time and it is also possible to test with ultrasonic bath extracts, as these can be ready within half an hour. Still, although patch testing with ultrasonic bath extracts is a simple technique, it is more laborious and time-consuming than testing with the materials as they are. The technique should, therefore, be used judiciously.

Table 12.1 Indications for the use of ultrasonic bath extracts

1. To avoid false-negative patch test reactions to a product/material
2. To avoid irritant reactions from a solid product/material
3. To get standardized patch test solutions for testing groups
4. To patch test controls
5. To patch test with thin-layer chromatograms
6. To perform chemical analyses based on patch-tested products/materials

12.6.1.1 To Avoid False-Negative Patch Test Reactions to a Product/Material

Many times it is sufficient to patch test a product/material as is in order to trace it to a contact allergy. However, sometimes this testing may be false negative and the undiagnosed contact allergy may yet be clinically relevant. This is particularly the case when the undiagnosed contact allergy to the product/material represents a weak contact allergy together with an extensive exposure to the product/material. Obviously, this situation occurs more frequently occupationally where a worker may handle a special product/material a hundred times a day, 5 days a week. In wet work or within hospital care, employees may use gloves many hours a day, 5 days a week. In these situations, with an extensive exposure to a contact sensitizer at a low concentration in a product/material to undamaged or damaged skin, the exposure may suffice to cause or significantly contribute to an allergic contact dermatitis on the hands, although the contact allergy to the product/material may be weak. In hospital personnel who wear gloves many hours a day, the testing with the gloves as they are may suffice but sometimes the testing with the gloves may be false negative. Recently, we published on glove dermatitis in hospital employees [8]. In 22 % of the employees with glove dermatitis, patch testing with an ultrasonic bath extract was needed to establish the diagnosis. Two other examples are given in which patch testing with ultrasonic bath extracts was necessary for the diagnosis of occupational allergic contact dermatitis. As demonstrated in the cases, patch testing with the objects as they are should always be performed when possible.

Case 1

A 33-year-old woman suffered from a severe atopic dermatitis and asthma/rhinitis since early childhood. Dermatologists and general practitioners had prescribed mainly topical corticosteroids and moisturizers for her skin. During these years she was never patch tested. In the 1980s she worked as a post office clerk with assignments that included a lot of handling of various types of papers such as forms and cartoons. When visiting the health department of the post office, the physician thought that it was strange that the dermatitis almost exclusively had been located to the hands and face during the last years. Because of this the patient was referred to the Department of Occupational Dermatology in Lund, where I was responsible for the investigation in the late 1980s. At examination a lichenoid dermatitis was seen on the face and hands. Nothing in the macroscopic morphology spoke against atopic dermatitis as the primary diagnosis. As an endogenous dermatitis can be significantly aggravated through exposure to exogenous hazardous factors, patch testing was performed with a baseline series and patient-supplied products including various paper forms, envelopes and cartons, as well as toiletries and cosmetics. These paper-based products were tested as they were and as ultrasonic bath extracts. Positive reactions were noted to methylchloroisothiazolinone/methylisothiazolinone (MCI/MI) and colophony in the baseline series. The various paper-based materials yielded negative reactions when tested as they were, whereas there were positive reactions to ultrasonic bath extracts of these materials.

In the late 1980s there was no legislation in Sweden requiring labeling of ingredients in toiletries and cosmetics. Because of the lack of labeling, we started in the mid of the 1980s to perform high-pressure liquid chromatography (HPLC) investigations of various types of products for the presence of MCI/MI in those who were hypersensitive to the preservative [9]. This preservative was detected in the cleansing cream that she used on the face every evening before going to bed. Because she was hypersensitive to various paper-based materials, she got different work assignments at the post office with substantially less exposure to paper-based materials and paper dust. At the same time she stopped using the facial cleansing cream containing MCI/MI, and these measures together with substantially less and no exposure to paper-based materials and cream, respectively, sufficed to virtually "heal" her dermatitis without any change in the topical treatment.

Case 2

A 35-year-old woman developed hand dermatitis, which was temporally related to her work. She worked at a plant renovating petrol engines. Her assignment was to assemble rubber-based gaskets on the engines. More than a hundred of these gaskets were handled manually daily. Patch testing with our baseline series including rubber chemicals such as thiurams, paraphenylenediamine-substituted rubber chemicals, and mercaptobenzothiazoles as well as the rubber gaskets as they were resulted in negative reactions. On the other hand, patch testing with ultrasonic bath extract of the rubber gaskets resulted in a positive reaction. With this knowledge, other work assignments were given to her without exposure to the rubber gaskets. Gradually, the hand dermatitis disappeared.

These cases represent two different situations where testing with the product/material resulted in negative reactions. The second case did not have any contact allergy to any of the sensitizers in the baseline series, while the first case, similarly to the hospital employees with glove dermatitis [8], also was allergic to chemicals that are possible ingredients of the products/materials to which she tested negatively when tested as they were. For many products, including rubber items, plastics objects, and textiles, it is usually very difficult, or even impossible, to get information on ingredients used for manufacturing of these products/materials. One possibility is to look chemically for the presence of these sensitizers in the products/materials as exemplified by the HPLC analysis of MCI/MI of the facial cream used by case 1. However, very few dermatologists have access to laboratories and indeed, there are no simple chemical methods available to show the presence of, for example, rubber sensitizers in rubber items. Therefore, the assessment of whether the exposure to a particular rubber object in a rubber-hypersensitive person is clinically relevant must often be based on the results of patch testing with the rubber objects tested as they are. Usually, a negative result is interpreted as there is no need for the patient to avoid the rubber object, although there are dermatologists who encourage their rubber-hypersensitive patients to avoid exposure to all rubber objects independently of the result of patch testing. This latter approach may be difficult to carry out in certain situations and may not be advisable in others. Sometimes there is a frequent occupational exposure to rubber objects that cannot be replaced with other materials, and the possibility to get a work-related dermatoses approved as an occupational dermatoses may also depend on the possibility of showing a particular sensitizer in a rubber object or hypersensitivity to this object.

12.6.1.2 To Avoid Irritant Reactions from a Solid Product/Material

Irritant factors are common causes of contact dermatitis. Sometimes the irritancy is mediated mechanically when the skin is exposed to products/materials such as certain plants, metal objects, mineral and textile fibers, and plastics that, for example, may have a sharp or needle-like surface. Obviously, these products/materials cannot be tested as they are without giving irritant skin reactions. Contact sensitizers may also be present in these products/materials. Even if the skin exposure to these irritant products/materials is limited to prevent an irritant reaction, a coexisting contact allergy may, with the limited exposure, still suffice to manifest as an allergic contact dermatitis. The patch test problem is solved using ultrasonic bath extracts for the testing.

12.6.1.3 To Get Standardized Patch Test Solution for Testing Groups

Sometimes there are outbreaks of suspected contact dermatitis in groups of individuals occupationally or non-occupationally. When a solid product/material is among the suspected agents causing the dermatitis, it is advisable and often easier to use an ultrasonic bath extract of the suspected product/material for patch testing. The testing can then be performed in a standardized way, enabling all tested individuals to be tested with the same potential sensitizer at the same dose. Recently, there were outbreaks of itching dermatitis and rhinitis among employees at three different work places in three different regions in Denmark with no relation between the work places and regions. However, in all three work places, a new type of carpet glued to the floor was suspected to be the cause of the health problems. Ultrasonic bath extracts were made of the carpet with and without glue for patch testing [10]. Because there were positive reactions to the ultrasonic bath extracts, these were also used for patch testing in controls [10].

12.6.1.4 To Patch Test Controls

Whenever there is a positive patch test reaction to a patient-supplied chemical or product/material tested as is or in a diluted form or as an ultrasonic bath extract, testing in controls has to be performed to substantially diminish the likelihood that the positive patch test reaction represents a false-positive reaction unless it is known that the test preparation tested is not an irritant. For statistical reasons, 20 dermatitis patients should be tested without any positive reactions to support the interpretation that the patch test reaction initiated the control testing represented an allergic reaction. Thus, the diagnostics of contact allergy and allergic contact dermatitis in cases 1 and 2 above were based on the findings of positive reactions to ultrasonic bath extracts without any positive reactions in the controls.

Sometimes the necessary testing in controls of a product/material carries certain problems. If a plant has given a positive reaction, it may be difficult to perform and guarantee an equivalent testing in all controls. In this situation, an ultrasonic bath extract of the plant will enable a standardized testing in the controls. First, the ultrasonic bath extract of the plant or another product/material should be tested in dilutions on the subject with a positive reaction. The lowest concentration of the ultrasonic bath extract yielding a positive reaction should subsequently be used for the testing in 20 controls. With this procedure, the risk of active sensitization of the controls will be minimized.

12.6.1.5 To Patch Test with Thin-Layer Chromatograms

The major indication to test with thin-layer chromatograms is to identify the contact sensitizer in a compound product/material to which an individual has tested positively [11]. The same ultrasonic bath extract of the product/material can, in addition to being used for the initial testing, also be used for testing in controls and for the preparation of thin-layer chromatograms for patch testing. Unlike the testing with ultrasonic bath extracts in controls where the lowest concentration of the ultrasonic bath extract elicits a positive reaction in the index subject, the highest concentration of ultrasonic bath extract should usually be used for the thin-layer chromatogram preparation. This approach has been used successfully many times in individual cases [12, 13] and in a group of individuals hypersensitive to disperse dyes, furniture, herbal teas, and oxidized hair dyes [14–17].

12.7   Demonstration of Exposure

12.7.1 To Perform Chemical Analyses Based on Patch-Tested Products/Materials

Besides a positive reaction to a product tested as is, there is sometimes also a positive reaction to a chemically defined sensitizer in the baseline patch test series or in an additional series or when the sensitizer has been tested separately. Is the chemically defined sensitizer present in the product/material? Often there is no information stating whether or not the chemically defined substance is present in the product/material. Chemical analysis can tell whether the sensitizer is present or not. When present, quantification of the sensitizer in the ultrasonic bath extract can help draw a conclusion on the clinical relevance of the exposure, particularly if the chemically defined sensitizer has been patch tested in serial dilutions down to a negative reaction.

12.8   How to Make Ultrasonic Bath Extracts

Instructions in bullet points below are given on how to make ultrasonic bath extracts. The equipment needed to make these extracts is simple and non-expensive. The sonicating device can be placed anywhere in a laboratory while the evaporation should take place in a well-ventilated area.

- Use approximately 50–100 cm^2 of the product/material for the extract. Register the measured or estimated used area (Fig. 12.1).
- Put the material into a glass jar.

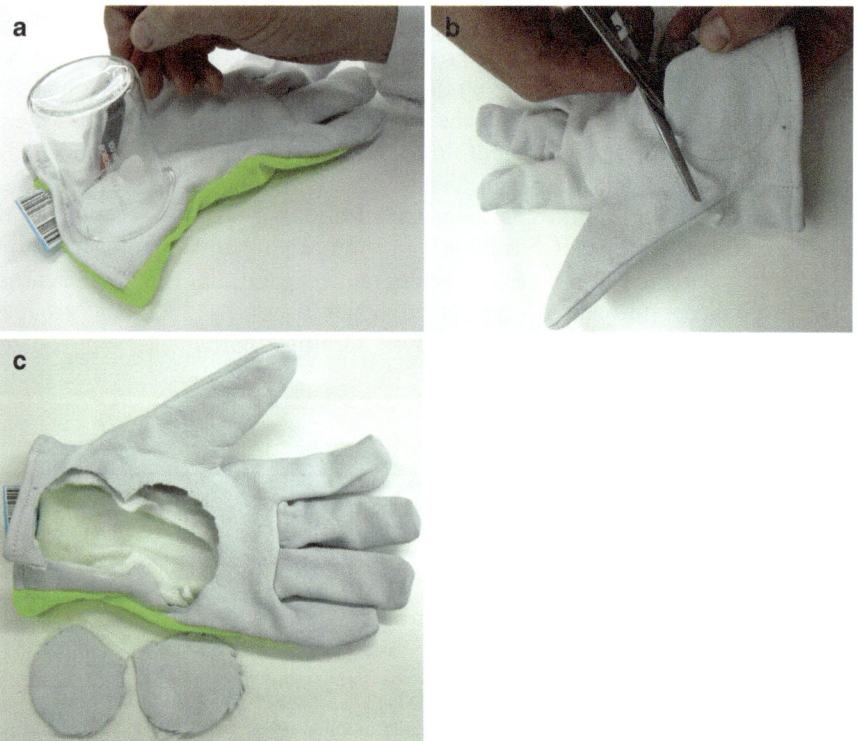

Fig. 12.1 (**a–c**) Use approximately 50–100 cm^2 of the product/material for the extract

Fig. 12.2 Add enough solvent to cover the product/material

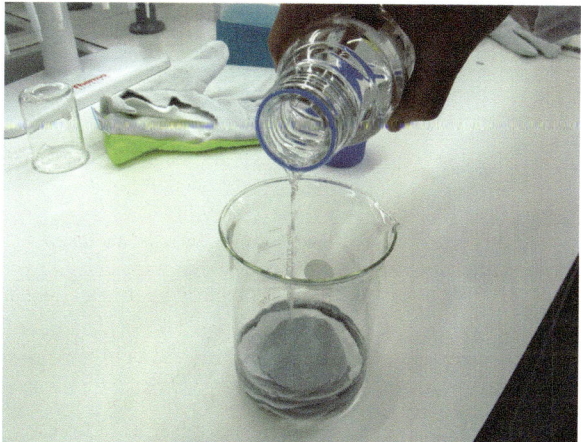

Fig. 12.3 Let the ultrasonic device be on for 5 min

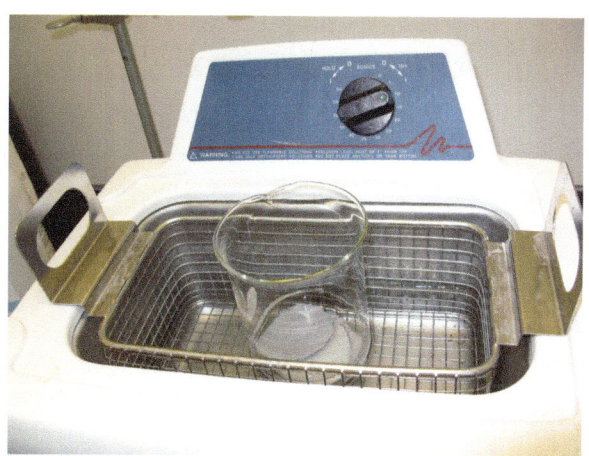

- Add enough solvent to the glass jar to cover the product/material. 5–20 mL is recommended. Register the type of solvent and volume used (Fig. 12.2).
- Let the ultrasonic device be on for 5 min (Fig. 12.3).
- Take away the solid product/material (Fig. 12.4).
- Let the extract evaporate to dryness. To speed up the evaporation, an evaporator can be used (Fig. 12.5). The evaporation should take place in a well-ventilated area.
- Add 1 mL of a skin-friendly solvent to the residue and transfer to a test tube. Make sure that the residue is dissolved (Fig. 12.6). This solution constitutes the stock solution, which can be tested as is and in dilutions, if desired.

Fig. 12.4 Take away the
solid product/material

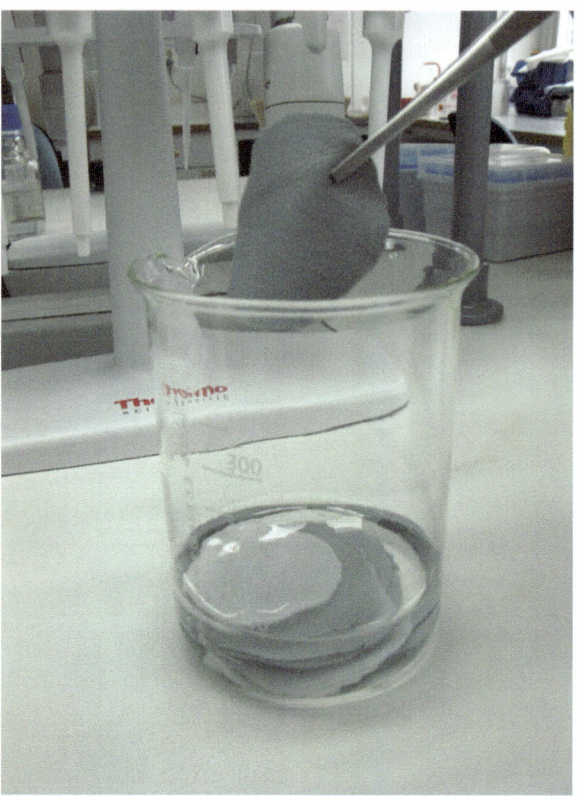

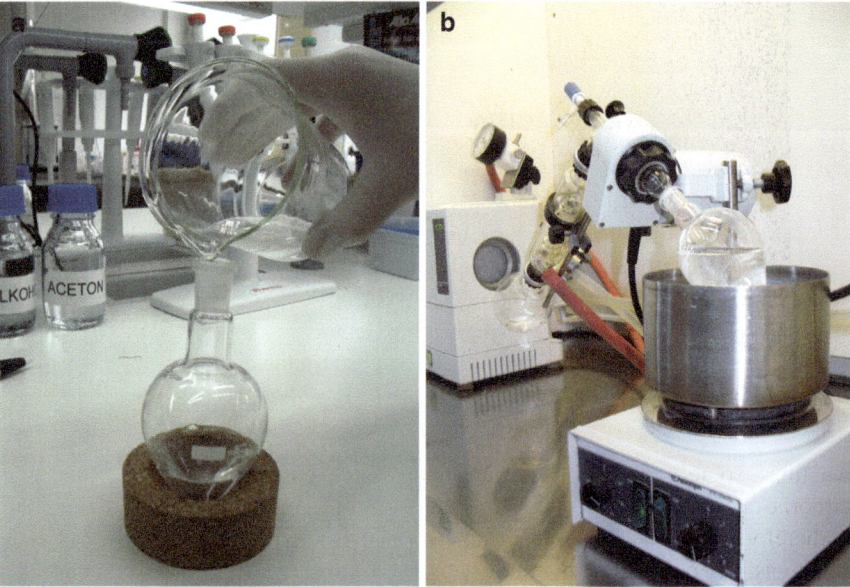

Fig. 12.5 (**a**, **b**) To speed up the evaporation, an evaporator can be used

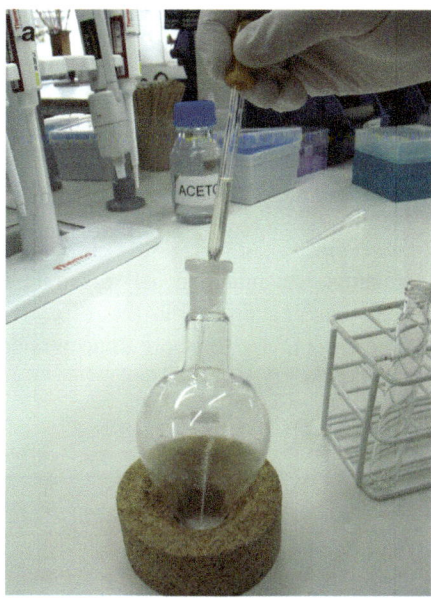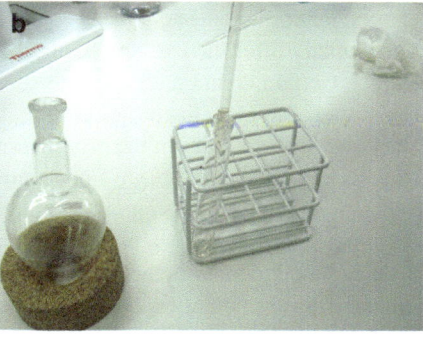

Fig. 12.6 (**a, b**) Add 1 mL of a skin-friendly solvent to the residue and transfer to a test tube. Make sure that the residue is dissolved

12.9 What Products/Materials to Be Tested?

Any solid product/material can be tested as an ultrasonic bath extract. We have used the technique for testing products such as rubber items, plastics objects, plants, wood, drugs, food items, concrete, textiles, clothes, shoes, metal objects, alloys, etc.

12.10 What Solvent Can Be Used to Make an Ultrasonic Bath Extract?

Any solvent can be used for the extraction. As always concerning chemical methods, environmentally friendly solvents should be preferred. Not all solvents are testable on the skin, but such solvents can still be used for the extraction provided that the solvent is completely evaporated after the extraction. A skin-friendly solvent can thereafter be used to make the final solutions for patch testing. Acidic and alkaline solvents can be used for extraction, but again, the final testing has to be done with a skin-friendly solvent within the recommended pH range [18]. It should be pointed out that the efficacy of the extraction procedure will vary with the sensitizer looked for, type of product/material, and extraction solvent. Acetone is the solvent predominantly used at our department. There are three major reasons for this: (1) it will extract both polar and nonpolar substances from the product/material, (2) it evaporates rapidly after the extraction, and (3) acetone is not irritating the skin at patch testing. Certain compounds, such as diphenylguanidine, are less soluble in acetone but more soluble in ethanol. Therefore, in situations where a particular sensitizer is suspected to be present in the product/material, the choice of solvent for the extraction should consider the physicochemical properties of the suspected sensitizer. When, for example, chromium in leather, concrete, or alloys is suspected, water will be used as extracting solvent. Occasionally, when there is a strong suspicion that a solid product/material is the cause of the dermatitis, we simultaneously make three different ultrasonic bath extracts with acetone, ethanol, and water as the respective solvent. Furthermore, it is, of course, possible to obtain even more concentrated extracts by adjustment of the various extraction factors.

12.11 Adverse Reactions

Like any test preparation, ultrasonic bath extracts may cause adverse reactions. According to my experience, irritant reactions are extremely rare. Still, whenever there is a positive reaction to an ultrasonic bath extract, a false-positive reaction due to irritancy may be the cause of the reaction why patch testing in controls should be considered. The most serious adverse reaction of patch testing is active sensitization. I have experienced this once 25 years ago when testing controls with an ultrasonic bath extract of a plant. After that occasion, controls are always patch tested with the lowest concentration of the ultrasonic bath extract eliciting a positive reaction in the index case.

Conclusion

Investigation of patients with suspected allergic contact dermatitis always requires patch testing with a baseline series but frequently also with additional series and patient-supplied products/materials. Many products/materials such as rubber items, plastics objects, plants, wood, drugs, food items, textiles, clothes, shoes, metal objects, and alloys can be tested as they are, but sometimes this testing can be false negative. The undiagnosed contact allergy can still be clinically relevant, particularly when the undiagnosed contact allergy to the product/material is weak and the exposure to the product/material is extensive. The idea behind patch testing with ultrasonic bath extracts is to test a possible but unknown contact sensitizer at a higher concentration than what is present in the product that has yielded a negative reaction when tested as is. The extraction procedure using an ultrasonic bath means an improved device to get standardized extracts from the same kind of products in a short time with regard to extraction area and time, volume of extracting solvent, use of ultrasonic bath, and evaporation, which enables the patient to be tested with extracts of patient-supplied products at the first visit to the patch test clinic. Besides the major indication to avoid false-negative patch test reactions to products/materials, ultrasonic bath extracts can be used for patch testing to avoid irritant reactions from a solid product/material, to get standardized solutions for testing groups of individuals, to test controls, to test with thin-layer chromatograms, and to perform chemical analyses based on patch-tested products/materials. Since the late 1980s we have tested thousands of ultrasonic bath extracts. In a low percentage of the patients tested with these extracts, positive reactions have exclusively been noted to the extracts. Subsequently, the revealed hypersensitivity and exposure to the product/material have been shown to be the major cause of the dermatitis [7, 10].

Practical Tips
- Patch test with ultrasonic bath extracts of solid products/materials when the exposure to the product/material is extensive.
- Patch test with ultrasonic bath extracts to avoid irritant reactions from a solid product/material.
- Patch test with ultrasonic bath extracts of products/materials to get standardized solutions for testing groups of individuals.

References

1. Bruze M. What it a relevant contact allergy? Contact Dermatitis. 1990;23:224–5.
2. Bruze M. Principles of occupational hand eczema. In: Menné T, Maibach HI, editors. Hand eczema. Boca Raton: CRC Press; 1993. p. 165–78.
3. Lachapelle J-M. Historical aspects. Chapter 1. In: Johansen JD, Frosch PJ, Lepoittevin J-P, editors. Contact dermatitis. 5th ed. Berlin: Springer; 2011. p. 1–9.
4. Peiser M, Tralau T, Heidler J, Api AM, Arts JHE, Basketter DA, et al. Allergic contact dermatitis: epidemiology, molecular mechanisms, in vitro methods and regulatory aspects. Cell Mol Life Sci. 2012;69:763–81.
5. Bruze M, Condé-Salazar L, Goossens A, Kanerva L, White IR. Thoughts on sensitizers in a standard patch test series. The European Society of Contact Dermatitis. Contact Dermatitis. 1999;41:241–50.
6. Bruze M, Gruvberger B, Björkner B. Kathon® CG – an unusual contact sensitizer. In: Menné T, Maibach HI, editors. Exogenous dermatoses: environmental dermatitis. Boca Raton: CRC Press; 1990. p. 283–98.
7. Bruze M, Trulsson L, Bendsöe N. Patch testing with ultrasonic bath extracts. Am J Contact Dermatitis. 1992;3:133–7.
8. Pontén A, Hamnerius N, Bruze M, Hansson C, Persson C, Svedman C, et al. Occupational allergic contact dermatitis caused by sterile non-latex protective gloves: clinical investigation and chemical analyses. Contact Dermatitis. 2013;68:103–10.
9. Gruvberger B, Persson K, Björkner B, Bruze M, Dahlquist I, Fregert S. Demonstration of Kathon CG in some commercial products. Contact Dermatitis. 1986;15:24–7.
10. Ebbehöj NE, Agner T, Zimerson E, Bruze M. Prevalence of eczema and rhinitis in a group of office-workers in Greenland (submitted).
11. Bruze M, Frick M, Persson L. Patch testing with thin-layer chromatograms. Contact Dermatitis. 2003;48:278–9.

12. Svedman C, Isaksson M, Zimerson E, Bruze M. Occupational contact dermatitis from a grease. Dermatitis. 2004;15:41–4.
13. Isaksson M, Zimerson E. Risks and possibilities in patch testing with contaminated personal objects: usefulness of thin-layer chromatograms in a patient with acrylate contact allergy from a chemical burn. Contact Dermatitis. 2007;57:84–8.
14. Lundh K, Gruvberger B, Möller H, Persson L, Hindsén M, Zimerson E, et al. Patch testing with thin-layer chromatograms of chamomile tea in patients allergic to sesquiterpene lactones. Contact Dermatitis. 2007;57:218–23.
15. Ryberg K, Goossens A, Isaksson M, Gruvberger B, Zimerson E, Persson L, et al. Patch testing of patients allergic to Disperse Blue 106 and Disperse Blue 124 with thin-layer chromatograms and purified dyes. Contact Dermatitis. 2009;60:270–8.
16. Lammintausta K, Zimerson E, Hasan T, Susitaival P, Winhoven S, Gruvberger B, et al. An epidemic of furniture-related dermatitis: searching for a cause. Br J Dermatol. 2010;162: 108–16.
17. Malinauskiene L, Zimerson E, Bruze M, Ryberg K, Isaksson M. Textile dyes disperse Orange 1 and Yellow 3 contain more than one allergen as shown by patch testing with thin-layer chromatograms. Dermatitis. 2011;22:335–43.
18. Bruze M. Use of buffer solutions for patch testing. Contact Dermatitis. 1984;10:267–9.

Patch Testing in the Tropics

13

Chee Leok Goh

13.1 Introduction

The tropical climate is hot and humid throughout the year. The ambient temperature is usually >25 °C and humidity >70 % throughout the year. There is very little seasonal variation. Patch testing in the tropics becomes a challenge to dermatologists because the application of occlusive patch test allergens with sticky tapes can cause discomfort to the patient, and adhesive tapes used for holding the test chambers in place often get displaced because of sweating. In this chapter, pitfalls and tips on patch testing in the tropics are presented.

13.2 Conducting Patch Testing Procedure in the Tropics

13.2.1 Ideal Patch Test Season

As there is little climatic variation through the year in the tropics, there is no ideal season to perform the patch test. Patch testing is carried out throughout the year. However, patch testing can be an uncomfortable procedure for the patients in the tropics because the ambient heat and high humidity cause sweating, making it difficult for adhesive tape to remain on the skin. Patients should be counseled about the procedure before it is carried out.

13.2.2 Ideal Patch Test System

The Finn chambers or the IQ chambers appear to be the most suitable patch test chambers for tropical use. Scanpore or Micropore tapes appear to be suitable

C.L. Goh, MD, MBBS, MMed (Int Med), MRCP(UK), FRCPE, FAMS
National Skin Centre, 1 Mandalay Road, Singapore 308205, Singapore
e-mail: drgohcl@gmail.com

J.-M. Lachapelle et al. (eds.), *Patch Testing Tips*,
DOI 10.1007/978-3-642-45395-3_13, © Springer-Verlag Berlin Heidelberg 2014

adhesive tapes in the tropics because they are strong and pliable and porous. The T.R.U.E. Test is also a suitable system for the tropics but is limited by its cost and limited range of allergens.

13.2.3 Patch Testing Procedure

The high ambient temperature and humidity in the tropics preclude some modification in our standard patch testing procedure.

1. Patients should be advised to cease all vigorous outdoor activities while undergoing the patch testing procedure. Those engaged in indoor duties should also be advised to remain in a cool and well-ventilated environment to minimize sweating.
2. Patients should be allowed to shower after application of the patch test chambers, but should be instructed to keep the patch test areas dry. The patient may be allowed to wipe the surrounding skin of patch test area with moist towels.
3. Patients should be advised to return to the clinic to reinforce the adhesive plaster when they are seen to be displaced.
4. After the removal of the chambers at 48 h, patients should be instructed to continue to keep the patch test area dry, but the surrounding skin can be cleaned with a moist towel, until the final patch test reading at 96 h.
5. Skin marking is preferably done with special marking inks. We found the preparation containing gentian violet 1 %, methyl alcohol 50 %, silver nitrate 20 %, and distilled water 29 % w/w to be most lasting. However, the preparation may cause skin irritation. Freshly prepared ink may be preferred, as the ink constituents become too concentrated as the solvent evaporates over time. Commercial skin markers and fluorescent markers do not stay long on the skin due to perspiration and humidity in the tropics.
6. For patients with dark skin, it may be necessary to examine the patch test area in a brightly lit room.

13.2.4 Occlusion Duration

In the tropics, it is preferred that the duration of the patch be as short as possible, as the adhesive tapes tend to get displaced because of sweating and thereby affect optimal occlusion. Ideally, patch testing is done on a Monday and reading done on the following Wednesday and Friday. Under such circumstances, it may be necessary to provide a medical certificate to the employer to exempt the patient from outdoor activities and/or strenuous activities for the first 3 days to ensure that the adhesive/test chamber remains in place.

A good alternative is to carry out the patch test over a weekend (e.g., on a Friday) so that the patient can remain indoors in a cooler environment at home. The patient can then be instructed to remove the patch test chambers themselves on a Sunday (after 48-h occlusion) and return on the following Monday (72-h reading) or on a

Tuesday (96-h reading). This will omit the 48-h reading. This protocol suits most patients very well in the hot and humid tropical climate without severely affecting their work.

There have been a few studies to ascertain if the duration of occlusion of patch test allergens can be shortened to less than 2 days' duration without affecting the diagnostic accuracy. However, the studies have indicated that although the overall concordance of results after 24 and 48 h of occlusion is high, clinically relevant allergens would have been missed if only the 24-h occlusion test was performed. In light of these results, it is recommended that the standard 48-h application remains appropriate for diagnostic patch testing [1].

13.2.5 Patch Test Reading

Most patients in the tropics have darker skin phototype, viz., skin types IV–VI. For patients with fair skin types II–IV, a positive patch test reaction is easy to identify. The erythema, papules, and mild edema and vesiculation are usually obvious. In the darker skin types V and VI, however, a mild positive allergic reaction may be overlooked as the erythema may not be visible. However, the edema, papules, and vesicles are usually discernible by palpation. Hence, when reading patch test reactions in dark-skinned individuals, it should be carried out in a well-lit room; palpation of the patch test site may help to detect features of an allergic patch test reaction.

13.2.6 Storage of Patch Test Allergen in the Tropics

Most of the patch test allergens are suspended in petrolatum as a vehicle. Petrolatum liquefies at high ambient temperature and affects the homogeneity of patch test allergen. In the tropics, where the ambient temperature is high, it is imperative that the patch test allergen tubes be stored in a cool place, preferably in a special refrigerator. In a study, it was found that nickel sulfate and potassium dichromate patch test materials become less homogeneous if stored at room temperature in a tropical country compared to storage at 4 °C. It would appear that the patch test materials should be stored in a refrigerator in between use when in the tropics [2].

13.3   Unique Contact Allergens in the Tropics

13.3.1 Topical Medicaments and Traditional Medicine

The prevalence and cause of allergic contact dermatitis vary in tropical countries. However, topical medicaments and herbal products are more commonly used in the tropics, especially in Asian countries [3]. Self-medication with over-the-counter (OTC) medicaments is a common practice in the tropics. Some of these

OTC remedies can cause contact allergy and should be considered for patch testing [4–6]. However, the exact ingredients of such OTC products are often unknown, making it difficult to ascertain the exact causative allergen in the allergic contact dermatitis. Well-known allergens include proflavine, nitrofurazone, tea tree oil, and Chinese herbal medication. These substances should be included for patch testing when investigating patients with suspected allergic contact dermatitis in the tropics.

13.3.2 Plant Dermatitis in the Tropics

In tropical Asia, a group of plants referred to locally as "rengas" are a common cause of allergic phytodermatitis. "Rengas" is a name derived by the indigenous people in Southeast Asia where the plants flourish. It consists of four genera of plants, namely, Gluta, Melanochyla, Melanorrhoea, Semecarpus, and Swintonia. All belong to the Anacardiaceae family. Injured bark of these plants secretes a toxic resinous sap that blackens when exposed to the air and becomes a resin that is notorious for causing allergic contact dermatitis. The chemical nature of this resin is unknown. It is believed to be a potent skin irritant and sensitizer. Carpenters and users of furniture are known to risk sensitization [7].

Exotic woods from tropical and subtropical regions such as South America, South Asia, and Africa (e.g., Dalbergia nigra [Rio rosewood] and Machaerium scleroxylon [Pao ferro]) frequently are used occupationally and recreationally by woodworkers and hobbyists. These exotic woods more commonly provoke irritant contact dermatitis reactions, but they also can provoke allergic contact dermatitis [8].

Another plant known to cause phytodermatitis in the tropics is the mango plant (*Mangifera spp.*). It too belongs to the Anacardiaceae family. Outbreaks of dermatitis from the plant saps often occur during the fruiting seasons. The allergen comes from the sap of the stem. The exact allergen remains unknown.

Clinicians must be aware of the potential for allergic contact dermatitis reactions to compounds in rengas plants, exotic woods, and mango saps. Patch testing should be performed with suspected woods and plant components for diagnostic confirmation.

13.3.3 Cosmetic Dermatitis

Characteristic allergic contact dermatitis in the tropics from cosmetics is seen in Hindu females who developed pigmented contact dermatitis from a red dye (kumkum) that is painted on their forehead. One of the causative allergens is Sudan I, which was previously reported to cause outbreaks of pigmented contact dermatitis in Japan. A similar practice of pasting red sticky paper on the forehead instead of the red dye powder has been reported to cause allergic contact dermatitis from the PTBP resins [9].

Practical Tips

- There are observed differences in the epidemiology of contact dermatitis in the tropics and temperate countries.
- Due to cultural differences, contact dermatitis from self-medication and use of herbal preparation is more common in the tropics, necessitating inclusion of these allergens for patch testing.
- The high ambient temperature and humidity in the tropics throughout the year exclude any ideal season for patch testing.
- Because of the high ambient temperature and humidity, some modification in the patch test procedures is required to ensure that the occlusive effects of patch testing are maintained and that patients comply with the procedure. Special markers and allowing patients to clean themselves are necessary.
- It is necessary to store patch test allergens in refrigerators in between use to maintain homogeneity of test allergens.

References

1. Ale SI, Maibach HI. 24-hour versus 48-hour occlusion in patch testing. Exog Dermatol. 2003;2:270–6.
2. Goh CL, Kwok SF. The influence of temperature on the concentration homogeneity of patch test materials. Contact Dermatitis. 1986;15:231–4.
3. Ng SK. Topical traditional Chinese medicine. A report from Singapore. Arch Dermatol. 1998;134(11):1395–6.
4. Lim KS, Tang MB, Goon AT, Leow YH. The role of topical traditional Chinese medicaments as contact sensitisers in chronic venous leg ulcer patients. Ann Acad Med Singapore. 2007;36(11):942–6.
5. Lee TY, Lam TH. Mastix is another allergen causing bone-setter's herbs dermatitis. Contact Dermatitis. 2001;44(5):312–3.
6. Lee TY, Lam TH. Allergic contact dermatitis due to a Chinese orthopaedic solution tieh ta yao gin. Contact Dermatitis. 1993;28(2):89–90.
7. Goh CL. Occupational contact dermatitis from Rengas wood. Contact Dermatitis. 1988; 18(5):300.
8. Podjasek JO, Cook-Norris RH, Richardson DM, Drage LA, Davis MD. Allergic contact dermatitis from exotic woods: importance of patch-testing with patient-provided samples. Dermatitis. 2011;22(2):E1–6.
9. Lilly E, Kundu RV. Dermatoses secondary to Asian cultural practices. Int J Dermatol. 2012; 51(4):372–9.

Contact Dermatitis in a Rapidly Changing Society: Experiences in Korea

14

Hee Chul Eun

14.1 Introduction

Contact dermatitis is closely related to environmental conditions and social status. Patch test remains essential in identifying causative materials producing contact dermatitis. However, patch test does suffer from limitations that can impede the final interpretation of the results and subsequent recommendations for patients regarding avoidance of causative agents, particularly in developing countries.

About a year ago, there was an article in an issue of Time magazine. This article claimed that since 1950 only Korea and Taiwan have maintained an average annual GDP growth rate of 5 % or more over the past 50 years, although six countries have maintained this rate of growth for four decades [1]. This suggests to us that contact dermatitis in Korea could be a good model for a rapidly changing society in a relatively short time.

This article addresses the difficulties and limitations of performing patch test in a developing country showing various experiences in Korea.

14.2 Limits of Patch Test

In principle, patch test is very simple. However, various factors can diminish the value of the final test results, which can be stressful to the performers. In countries where information gathering and patients' referral system are relatively good for the dermatologists, patch test can be attractive. However, in many countries the situation is the opposite, because of the following factors, which I would like to mention in detail.

H.C. Eun, MD, PhD
Department of Dermatology, Seoul National University Hospital,
101, Daehang-ro, Jongno-gu, Seoul 110-744, Republic of Korea
e-mail: hceun@snu.ac.kr

J.-M. Lachapelle et al. (eds.), *Patch Testing Tips*,
DOI 10.1007/978-3-642-45395-3_14, © Springer-Verlag Berlin Heidelberg 2014

14.2.1 Reproducibility

Patch test is an in vivo test. Therefore, many unknown factors may affect the final patch test result. The possible factors related to the false-positive and false-negative reactions of patch test were already well described about 40 years ago by Sultzburger [2]. Compared to the time of his report, standardization of test methods has improved quite a bit. Despite this improvement, poor reproducibility of patch test remains a serious problem, which was shown well by Gaullhausen et al. [3]. In the report, if we perform the same test on the same individuals using the Finn Chambers system, nearly 40 % of the positive results were not reproducible at the sequential testing, and 43.8 % were nonreproducible at concomitant testing. The author also pointed out that weakly positive reactions are far more often nonreproducible than stronger reactions [3]. Even if using TRUE test, the most up-to-date system of patch test, 17.9 % of tests results are not reproducible [4]. This means that from the applying antigens to the final reading of the test results, many delicate factors may be involved. Therefore, the true meaning of patch test reactions needs cautious interpretation.

Patch testing is not usually recommended in patients with active skin lesions because of the possibility of false-positive reaction. However, for practical reasons dermatologists cannot always perform patch test in the complete absence of patients' skin lesions. It means that false-positive reaction due to the existing dermatitis can affect the patch test reaction all the time. As there is currently no other appropriate alternative diagnostic test for patients with contact dermatitis, patch test should be done carefully according to the guidelines to maximize reproducibility.

14.2.2 Antigens and Cost

Many commercial patch test antigens should be imported from other countries. This increases the cost of patch test, which can be relatively expensive. In addition to the frequently used standard antigens, other antigens that are rarely used are also required. However, the consumption rate is very low in many institutes if they do not test enormous numbers of cases annually. These rare antigens may not be stably maintained in storage considering their scant use. Therefore, a reasonable rate of use would be required in terms of the cost and the stability. Moreover, in many countries, including Korea, patients must pay a portion or the full cost of the test fee, which is another burden to the simultaneous testing of many antigens. In Korea only 30 antigens are covered by the national insurance. Testing involving more antigens is directly billed to the patients.

Additional antigens that are not commercially available can be difficult to prepare in terms of time and energy. Therefore, many dermatologists usually use the standard battery only, which is another reason that the test results are not so productive to make a final conclusion. In this sense, referral of testing to an accredited hospital that has access to numerous antigens may be desirable, although this option may not be readily available in many developing countries. For example, in Korea hospitals competitively care for patients, with doctors paid according to the number of the patients they care for. Therefore, doctors do not want to refer patients to other hospitals for additional patch testing except in cases that might otherwise involve legal disputes.

14.2.3 Information and Medical System

Dermatologists who perform patch tests need information related to the suspected antigens or materials. However, access to information can be limited, especially in developing countries. Even in developed countries, information may be restricted due to proprietary interests of vendors. Getting information is the first step to verify the patient's problem; however, its approach is very much limited according to the social and medical system. With active use of the Internet, the capabilities of reference search and obtaining information have improved compared with the past. However, even though information and relevant additional materials are available to the dermatologists, it is a really challenging and time-consuming work to verify the final causative agents. In addition, patients may be reluctant to undergo retesting with the individual ingredients that have required considerable time and energy for preparation.

14.2.4 Relevance and Interpretation

A negative patch test can be a relief to the dermatologists, since it ends the search for a source of dermatitis. However, a positive patch test can prompt an arduous search for the source of dermatitis. Although certain semiquantitative scoring systems may be helpful for the evaluation of relevance, as Lachapelle mentioned [5], its level of application can vary considerably among dermatologists of different countries. Various factors such as good clinical data, environmental evaluation, acquiring information, and analysis are vital to increase the relevant scoring. However, these activities can be onerous for busy physicians who are not working under a specialized and well-designed system. This means that individual tracing of perfect relevance is not always satisfactory even in a developed society with more resources and facilities, which is another big challenge of performing patch test. There is no doubt that dermatologists in developing countries are much more likely to face this kind of difficulties.

14.2.5 Prognosis

After a patch test, a patient's skin trouble may not be relieved effectively, even when contact with relevant antigens or irritants is avoided. Some antigens are ubiquitous, and it may be the source of the persisting skin trouble. However patients' skin lesions sometimes persist even though complete avoidance has seemingly been achieved. It is also well known that in contact dermatitis due to some industrial antigens, such as chrome, the prognosis is relatively poor, even after avoidance of the causative agent or a job change [6]. Sometimes complicated legal problems can appear, and the potential legal ramification can dissuade dermatologists from caring for patients with industrial-related problems.

14.3   Experiences in Korea

Despite the aforementioned negative aspects of patch testing, I would like to emphasize that dermatologists in a developing country should more actively use patch test as a means of safeguarding people from emerging and perhaps little-recognized hazardous agents. In cases in which we are searching well-known agents in a society, it may be easy to diagnose the culprits. However, unfamiliar agents producing dermatitis are very difficult to identify without painstaking hard work by the physicians.

Korea, one of the poorest countries in the world only about 50 years ago, has been transformed into a high-tech society. Therefore, it may be worthwhile to review various experiences in this country as a model of contact dermatitis in a developing society. With this in mind, some examples were introduced with a few practical and important ideas concerning patch test and contact dermatitis.

14.3.1 General Medical System in Korea

A necessary and important prelude to a discussion of contact dermatitis and patch test is an understanding of the general medical system of the country of concern, in this case Korea, since this will affect the performance of the patch test in various ways. The Korean medical insurance system was initially adopted from Japan in the late 1970s, but the major difference in Korea today is that it is totally controlled by one government institute. Every worker pays 5.3 % of their average income as an insurance fee, with half covered by employers. It is basically a partial coverage system. For example, the admission fee is covered at 80 % from insurance, while outpatient fees are covered at only 50 %. It is more favorable for children (90 % coverage) and for extremely poor persons who receive a complete deduction. The medical fee is inexpensive and under socialized control by the government. Since the fee is seldom increased, doctors must see many patients to match the revenue. Large hospitals are allowed to operate other related businesses such as funeral homes and restaurants to compensate for the financial burden. The greatly discounted medical insurance system in Korea contrasts with full-coverage systems in many western countries. One of the key factors worth mentioning in Korea is that the government has not invested much in hospital facilities except for regional public health centers whose roles include vaccination and control of venereal diseases, as two examples. Most hospital facilities are funded by private institutes or individuals. This system did work relatively well. But in a time when increasing numbers of hospitals are facing financial problems, discontent with the government's monopoly of medical fee control is growing. And this conflict is getting worse due to the rapid increase of aging population, which is a great burden to the medical insurance system year by year.

14.3.2 Industrial Dermatology

One of the attractive points in the field of contact dermatitis is industrial dermatology. This is because every factory can be a good research model. Occupational dermatoses are frequently neglected even in a developed society because doctors, as well as workers, regard them as non-life-threatening conditions. Excluding some developed nations, the system does not favor dermatologists. As the systems of diagnosis, management, and compensation for industrial dermatology vary between different countries, the reporting systems are also different.

An annual routine special medical examination is the key system of managing industrial diseases in Korea and is performed by doctors of preventive medicine. These physicians are very wary of friction with the industrial companies who pay the examination fees and can change the institutes. Doctors involved in special examination generally lack clinical experiences of skin diseases. They do not want to change the present system that is oriented towards preventive medicine. They are very ambivalent to mass media reports of industrial diseases. Sometimes they acknowledge them when they appear in the headlines of newspapers, but they are afraid of them in many cases, especially when the report occurs in their operating zone. They are occasionally interested in skin research, which sometimes gives dermatologists the opportunity to participate in a certain project.

The Korean government does not want occupational diseases to appear as major issues on mass communication and has adopted a passive stance about compensation of occupational skin diseases. Officers in the labor department know the problem of managing the system of occupational skin diseases in general, but are passive in reformation. They are satisfied with low reports of occupational skin diseases in general.

Dermatologists in Korea are reluctant to care for occupational disease cases because of their already high workload and fear of legal disputes. Site visits, material analysis, and chemical information are usually not available. In addition, even though they spend much time in diagnosing occupational skin diseases, the effort is not rewarded with appropriate additional fees. Some dermatologists, including the author, are interested in limited research because many factories have their own peculiar research interests. However, fruitful results are relatively rare.

Although official reports of occupational skin disease are rare in Korea, a field survey will typically reveal a lot of occupational dermatoses without difficulty. In the early 1980s, the author surveyed in a certain industrial area as a member of a special medical examination team. Out of 4,325 industrial workers working in a hazardous environment, there were nearly 1.2 % cases of contact dermatitis [7]. As the system of diagnosis and management of occupational skin diseases has not changed much since then, similar findings would be anticipated today. One of the interesting points to mention is the perception that cases of industrial dermatoses are decreasing a little bit nowadays in Korea because many small factories with hygienic problems prone to producing occupational skin diseases have already relocated to other countries, such as China and Southeast Asia.

Dermatologists and physicians interested in industrial medicine have tried several times to change the legislation related to industrial medicine. However the government has been stubborn to change. Therefore, it is our recommendation that a joint approach, with sophisticated tactics by dermatologists, may be more successful for the ideal setting of medical system or industrial medicine in a developing country, if the government is interested in new policies related to this field. It is because as long as we do not have a reasonable system effective for diagnosis of contact dermatitis, the patch test will remain far from being of practical help.

14.3.3 Organizing National Contact Dermatitis Research Group

Since the foundation of the International Contact Dermatitis Research Group, many national and international contact dermatitis research groups have been organized. Although the levels of activities are various, a national contact dermatitis research group in a developing country can achieve some positive results, which include:
• Stimulating reports important to their societies
• Stimulating joint studies about subjects peculiar to their societies
• Sharing information of the contact sources important to their societies
• Spurring improvements in the relevant legal system

The Korean Contact Dermatitis Research Group was founded in 1980. Since then, through annual meetings, many reports have been presented and some of them published mainly in domestic journals.

In 1995 the author reviewed around 200 Korean references related to epidemiology and clinical aspects of contact dermatitis published for the past 20 years [8]. Table 14.1 summarizes the findings and various aspects of contact dermatitis profiles. Reports related to medicaments were relatively common, while reports related to cosmetics and occupation were relatively scant. This suggested that it was relatively easy to get information from the pharmaceutical companies, while cosmetics at that time were not labeled and diagnosis and management of occupational

Table 14.1 Reported papers related to epidemiology and clinical aspects of contact dermatitis in Korea

Items	No. of papers
General incidence	13
Routine patch tests	13
Plants, animals	25
Occupation	33
Medicaments	53
Cosmetics	23
Metals	19
Others	15
Total	194

Reprinted with permission from Eun [8]

dermatitis were poor. Unfortunately, the trend has persisted despite efforts of dermatologists to change the system related to patch test. At the present time, cosmetics are labeled; however, getting individual ingredients from cosmetic companies remains difficult, which hinders dermatologists from performing patch testing with individual ingredients because of the cost-effectiveness.

14.3.4 Standard Battery

The joint research of hospital prevalence data is always a useful indicator in any society, since it occupies nearly half of the causative agents showing positive patch test reactions. Table 14.2 shows the serial interval change of the most common allergens in Korea [9]. For instance, nickel sulfate continuously increased for the past 30 years, while chromate has recently decreased. Fragrance-related allergens such as fragrance mix and Balsam of Peru have shown a decreasing tendency. For some antigens, such as thimerosal and para-tertiary butylphenol formaldehyde resin, it is

Table 14.2 Comparison of common standard allergens with previous KCDRG study (%)

Allergen	KCDRG (1983–1985) $N=937$	KCDRG (1986–1993) $N=2,326$	Present study (2009–2010) $N=795$
Nickel sulfate	12.9	17.9	34.1
Thimerosal	6.7	5.7	12.6
Cobalt chloride	NA	13.8	11.1
P-Phenylenediamine	7.3	3.4	8.4
P-tert Butylphenol formaldehyde resin	1.0	2.4	6.2
Potassium dichromate	11.8	11.3	5.6
Carba mix	NA	1.4	5.6
Fragrance mix	NA	12.9	5.2
Colophony	NA	3.3	4.3
Thiuram mix	3.2	2.6	3.7
Black rubber mix	2.7	1.0	3.5
Epoxy resin	1.2	2.5	3.3
Wool alcohols	3.0	3.3	2.9
Kathon CG	NA	NA	2.9
Neomycin sulfate	7.6	7.2	2.6
Balsam of Peru	7.0	4.7	2.6
Paraben mix	3.4	2.5	2.5
Formaldehyde	4.4	4.8	2.4
Quaternium 15	2.9	1.9	2.1
Caine mix	NA	NA	2.0
Ethylenediamine dihydrochloride	1.4	1.3	1.7
Mercapto mix	2.3	2.2	1.7
Mercaptobenzothiazole	NA	NA	1.5
Quinolone mix	NA	1.8	1.3

Reprinted with permission from Hong et al. [9]
Abbreviations: *KCDRG* Korean Contact Dermatitis Research Group, *NA* not available

very difficult to find the relevance. This type of research is most important to screen the prevalent allergens in their own society and can recruit more patients in a relatively short period of time. It is desirable to do joint research at regular intervals to find a serial change of a standard battery composed of common antigens suitable to their own societies.

Rhus is a very common antigen in many societies. However, it is not usually included in the standard battery because of its high risk of active sensitization. It was suggested that contact dermatitis due to Rhus plants seems to be decreasing owing to rapid urbanization [10]. However, in Korea systemic contact dermatitis due to Rhus ingestion is still problematic, since people are fond of eating Rhus with chicken to treat gastrointestinal disorders as well as a health food [11]. Nearly half of the patients have maculopapular drug eruption like rash; however, various rashes such as erythroderma, erythema multiforme, purpura, pustule, and wheals can appear. Considering the varieties of onset and some abnormal laboratory findings, several other mechanisms may be involved in addition to immunoallergic mechanism [11]. The main Rhus plant in Korea is *Rhus verniciflua* (Japanese lacquer tree), which is different from the species common in other societies such as poison ivy and poison sumac [12]. Cases with contact dermatitis from plants and animals are worth investigating in every country because a unique profile can be found in each society.

14.3.5 Rare Sporadic Case Reports

Rare clinical reports should not be overlooked, but rather considered as important, since they suggest that concurrent similar cases may exist in the particular societies. Even if the investigation is not perfect in a certain case, publication in relevant domestic journals should be encouraged. It is because the fully verified information can be difficult to obtain and patch testing with individual ingredients is not easy to perform in a developing country. Even if such clinical reports are not published in a domestic journal, recording such cases with abstracts is useful for the physicians. Also, it would be prudent for contact dermatitis researchers to establish an Internet presence, since this would facilitate contact with fellow researchers. There is no doubt that more sophisticated research of the same subject is needed for further information in detail.

Once someone has published a journal article, other authors will tend not to publish similar papers unless they involve many cases or a special investigation. Therefore, we should bear in mind that even one case may be important in representing a problem that is producing contact dermatitis at a certain period of time in a society.

Sometimes cases that occur in a domestic setting may have originated because of contact with dermatitis sources encountered during travel in a foreign country. Because native dermatologists are not used to this kind of problem, it is necessary to inform dermatologists worldwide of such cases, because it could be very helpful in diagnosing concurrent cases. Usually animals or plants encountered during travel are frequent culprits of contact dermatitis. Contact dermatitis due to jellyfish in Korea that occurred during travel in Southeast Asia is a good example [13]. This kind of problem increases according to the rapid increase of domestic GDP.

14.4   International Cooperation

14.4.1   Information Search

Nowadays information related to contact dermatitis is usually searched for with the aid of a computer; however, we still need some kind of useful connection between physicians with the same interests in different countries. In addition, it is necessary for dermatologists to set up their own information systems to record and share information that is unique to their countries.

14.4.2 Allergen Bank

Rare allergens are quite problematic in preparations that dermatologists make themselves in patch test clinics. Therefore, in many clinics, patch tests are usually performed either with standard series only or with several additional special batteries that are commercially available. In 1996, Andersen proposed a new concept of allergen bank to solve this problem. Through this system, rare antigens can be supplied to the physicians by central control [14]. However, this method needs a controlling system, and it will also face problems of delivery, storage, quality control, waiting time, and cost. As many allergens are commercially available nowadays, it may be better to use commercial antigens, although these are expensive. Notwithstanding this, the allergen bank system still could be worthwhile to operate regionally if it can be supported by someone outside. However, it may still be difficult for the physicians to use the resources owing to constraints of time, cost, and delivery.

14.4.3 Cooperative Step Against Regulation

The safety of patch test antigens is another concern. Many governments, including Korea, are striving to ensure tight control of antigen quality and safety, especially new antigens. The Food and Drug Administration wants to verify the safety of patch tests by determining whether patch test antigens are drug or diagnostic agents. In either case, the safety issue is unavoidable because patch test antigens penetrate and are absorbed by the human body, leading to the small possibility of potential health hazard. This will be a great challenge in the future for performing patch tests. Therefore, a global cooperative approach between different contact dermatitis research groups will be necessary in this regard.

14.4.4 Sharing Educational Model

Dermatologists in many developing countries still lack enough experience in handling agents that cause contact dermatitis. This will be improved by communication between dermatologists in different countries interested in contact dermatitis and patch tests. Establishment of a practically effective national educational system would be valuable. In addition, benchmarking of other countries' models may be necessary.

Conclusion

This review highlights the limitations and problems of patch test and presents some experiences in Korea. The author hopes this information will be helpful for dermatologists in developing countries to set their own system that will prove useful for better diagnosis and management of contact dermatitis.

Practical Tips
- Although patch test is still essential for diagnosis and management of contact dermatitis, it has limitations and disadvantages that hinder its use.
- As patch test is closely related to and affected by the society and its medical system, many dermatologists are not so satisfied with the final test results, especially in developing countries.
- Despite negative aspects of patch testing, dermatologists in a developing country should more actively use patch test as a means of safeguarding people from emerging and perhaps little-recognized hazardous agents.
- Korea is one of the fastest growing countries in the world, and review of the past experiences related to contact dermatitis could be useful in establishing a model for a developing country.
- Several ideas worthwhile to stress were illustrated: organization of national contact dermatitis research group, regular joint research, importance of rare cases, and a few strategies of international cooperation.

References

1. Sharma R. Hitting the brick wall. Time 2012 April 23, p. 40–44.
2. Sultzburger MB. The patch test- who should and should not use it and why. Contact Dermatitis. 1975;1:117–9.
3. Gallhausen R, Przybilla B, Ring J. Reproducibility of patch test. J Am Acad Dermatol. 1989; 21:1196–202.
4. Gollhausen R, Prizybilla B, Ring J. Reproducibility of patch test results: comparison of TRUE test and Finn Chamber test results. J Am Acad Dermatol. 1989;21:843–6.
5. Lachapelle JM. A proposed relevance scoring system for positive allergic patch test reactions: practical implications and limitations. Contact Dermatitis. 1997;36:39–43.
6. Goh CL. Hand eczema in the construction industry. In: Menné T, Maibach HI, editors. Hand eczema. 2nd ed. Boca Raton: CRC Press; 2000. p. 287–94.

7. Eun HC, Oh CW, Kye YC, Lim SK, Kim SN, Kim KC, et al. Study on occupational dermatoses in industrial workers. J Korean Med Assoc. 1982;25(6):552–60 [Korean].
8. Eun HC. Epidemiological and clinical review of contact dermatitis in Korea. Korean J Dermatol. 1995;33(2):209–24 [Korean].
9. Hong YJ, Choi HY, Kim KJ, Lee GY, Kim DW, Kim SJ, et al. TRUE test in patients with contact dermatitis: a multicenter study. Korean J Dermatol. 2011;49(8):661–9 [Korean].
10. Park KB, Eun HC, Lee YS. A study of the prevalence of contact sensitization to Rhus and gingko antigens. Korean J Dermatol. 1986;24(1):21–7 [Korean].
11. Park SD, Won TH. Systemic contact dermatitis due to Rhus. In: Eun HC, Kim SC, Lee WS, editors. Asian skin and skin diseases. Seoul: Mederang Inc; 2011. p. 65–71.
12. Eun HC, Kim MG, Kim SN. Epidemiological study of possible Korean plants involved in contact dermatitis. Korean J Dermatol. 1979;17(4):265–82 [Korean].
13. Park BC, Hough D, Kim HO, Kim CW. A case of delayed cutaneous reaction caused by jellyfish. Korean J Dermatol. 1991;29(2):214–7 [Korean].
14. Andersen KE, Rastoqi SC, Carlsen L. The allergen bank: a source of extra contact allergens for the dermatologists in practice. Acta Derm Venereol. 1996;76(2):136–40.

Immediate-Type Testing: Immunologic Contact Urticaria and Immunologic Contact Urticaria Dermatitis

15

Jessica A. Schweitzer and Howard I. Maibach

We note a relative paucity of literature on immunologic contact urticaria and protein contact dermatitis (now preferentially neologized-immunologic contact urticaria dermatitis). We find this term clearer than protein contact dermatitis, as the morphology is dermatitis, but the mechanism is IgE mediated. This brief chapter updates and simplifies testing algorithms in hopes of increasing their use.

Contact urticaria presents as a wheal and flare response that occurs within a few minutes to an hour or so of exposure to a substance absorbed by the skin [1]. Contact urticaria can be divided into three categories: immunologic contact urticaria (ICU), nonimmunologic contact urticaria (NICU), and uncertain mechanism-mediated contact urticaria [1]. NICU is the most common type and can occur without previous sensitization to a particular allergen. The wheal and flare are thought to occur with the substance directly affecting the vessels of the dermis or when vasoactive substances are released through a non-antibody-mediated pathway [1]. NICU does not produce systemic reaction such as anaphylaxis.

In contrast, ICU is mediated by an IgE type 1 hypersensitivity reaction and requires previous exposure and sensitization to a specific substance [2]. This type is rarer among the population, but it is more common in atopic individuals and their families [2]. Contact urticaria can manifest in any of the four clinical stages and can be considered a syndrome, as it affects many other organs besides the skin [1]:

Cutaneous Reactions Only

Stage 1: Localized urticaria, itching, burning, stinging, dermatitis

Stage 2: Generalized urticaria

Extracutaneous Reactions

Stage 3: Bronchial asthma, rhinoconjunctivitis, orolaryngeal symptoms, gastrointestinal symptoms

Stage 4: Anaphylactoid reactions

J.A. Schweitzer, BS (✉) • H.I. Maibach, MD, PhD
Department of Dermatology, University of California-San Francisco,
90 Medical Center Way, Surge 110, San Francisco, CA 94143-0989, USA
e-mail: jschweitzer09@gmail.com; maibachh@derm.ucsf.edu

J.-M. Lachapelle et al. (eds.), *Patch Testing Tips*,
DOI 10.1007/978-3-642-45395-3_15, © Springer-Verlag Berlin Heidelberg 2014

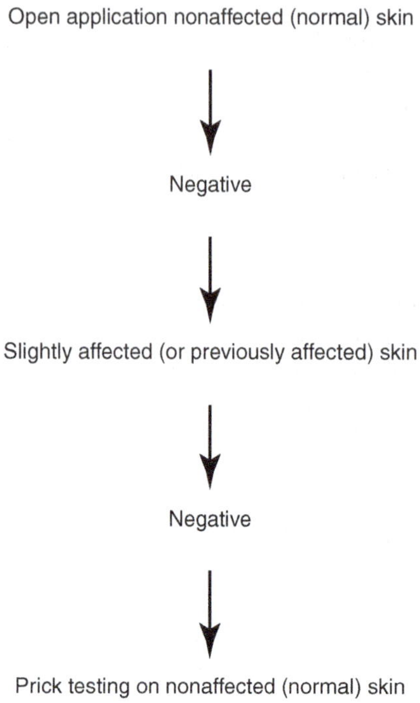

Fig. 15.1 Algorithm for contact urticaria testing

Open application nonaffected (normal) skin

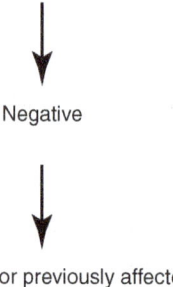

Negative

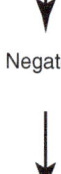

Slightly affected (or previously affected) skin

Negative

Prick testing on nonaffected (normal) skin

Fig. 15.2 Open and prick testing guidelines

Open and prick testing

- Open application
  - Normal skin
  - Slightly damaged skin
  - Atypical anatomic site
- If positive, either ICU, NICU, or ICUD
  - Control needed to verify if ICU or NICU
- Prick testing
  - Normal skin only
  - If positive, control needed to verify if ICU, NICU, or ICUD

The ideal test to perform first for evaluation of contact urticaria is open application of the suspected allergen on nonaffected skin and, if negative results ensue, on slightly affected skin (Fig. 15.1). If this does not elicit a response, then the prick test may be used. Note that certain anatomic sites such as the face are more reactive than the volar forearm [3]. In patients with mainly facial lesions, the product/chemical may be applied there if the forearm fails to reveal a positive result (Fig. 15.2).

Because the severity of each stage differs, it is important to elicit from a patient's history if they have had extracutaneous manifestations in the past with an allergen or when being tested with one. It is also advisable to perform the test in a setting that

Fig. 15.3 Positive prick test on normal skin (Reprinted with permission from Lachapelle and Maibach [4])

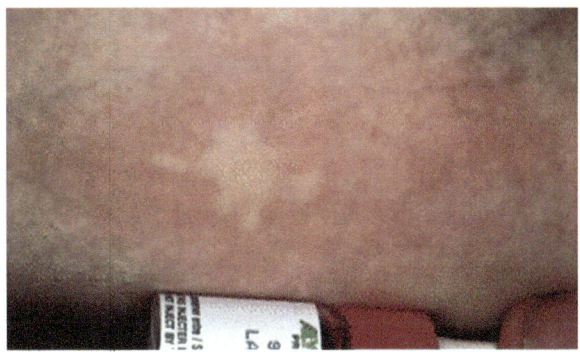

has the resources to treat a severe reaction. Fortunately, the prick test is a safer method to use than the scratch or intradermal test because a smaller dose is introduced into the skin.

When we first started ICU testing, we produced anaphylaxis (stage 4) by utilizing too high a concentration in open application testing (see Fig. 15.1). Hence, with chemical exposure eliciting systemic signs and symptoms, we start with serial dilutions. A simple time-efficient method consists of tenfold dilutions in physiologic saline (when soluble) and diluting 1:10 up to approximately 10^6. This can be done in the office with a dropper.

To perform the prick test, apply drops of the allergen solution on the upper back or volar forearm. Separate each allergen by 3.5 cm so as not to evoke a cross-reaction, and start with a low dilution to avoid a severe response [4]. If controls are needed, histamine chlorohydrate solution (10 mg/mL) or codeine phosphate solution (9 %) can be used. Codeine phosphate solution has a more uniform response [4]. However, anything that produces a wheal and flare on normal skin does not need a control unless the chemical produces NICU. The area can then be pricked with a lancet, and the skin should be examined for a positive response characterized by at least a 3-mm wheal or half the size of the control reaction after 15–30 min [5] (Fig. 15.3). The patient should stay on the premises for at least 30 min after the test to watch for an adverse response.

Some patients who work in the food industry and many others may encounter multiple allergens in their daily work. When a patient comes with this issue, advise the following:
- Make a list of all foods/chemicals that cause burning, stinging, or itching, as follows:
  1. Carrot
  2. Potato
  3. Salmon
  4. Kiwi
  5. Flour
  6. Milk
  7. Shrimp
- Have someone other than the patient place each type of food/chemical in question into separate small plastic bags, or place each type of food in an ice cube tray (Fig. 15.4).

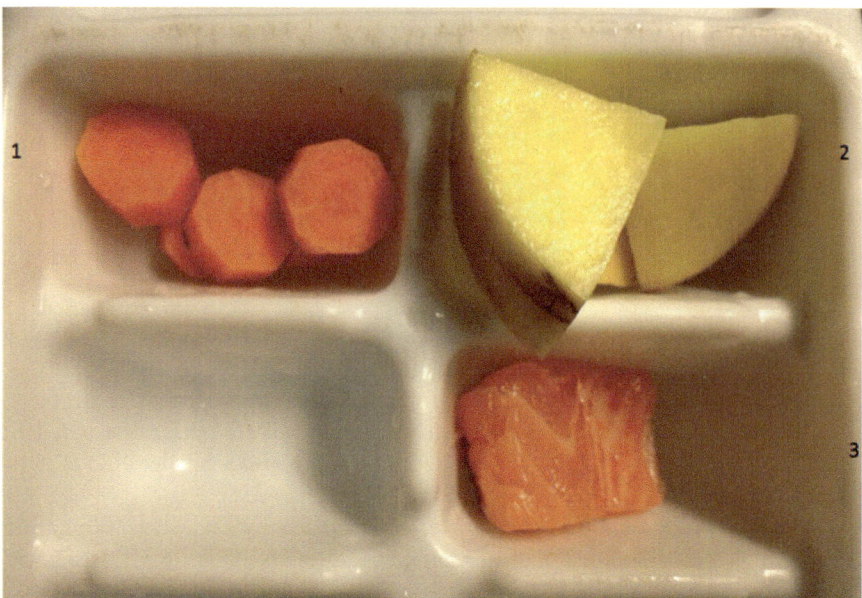

Fig. 15.4 Numbered ice cube tray filled with food/chemical corresponding to patient-made list

- Number the bags or each ice cube compartment, and match the number to the previous list made. Etain Cronin originally suggested this strategy.

In our experience, testing with commercially available food allergens generally induces a false negative, perhaps because of protein denaturation in heat or chemical processing/preservation, hence our use of fresh product/chemical.

Prick testing is an important and often underutilized tool in medicine. Some dermatologists may avoid it if they were not exposed to the procedure during their training, or they defer to allergists for the test to be performed. However, allergists are less likely to perform prick testing with natural products rather than preprepared commercial allergens, as the former are generally more time-consuming.

Practical Tips
- Use prick testing to diagnose ICU if open application testing on normal and affected skin fails to produce a positive response.
- Have the patient make a list of each food/chemical that causes symptoms and then have someone other than the patient place each food/chemical in separate plastic bags or ice cube tray compartments to bring into the office for testing.
- Using a dropper, dilute the suspected allergen beginning with tenfold dilutions in physiologic saline (when soluble) and diluting 1:10 up to approximately 10^6.

- The best areas to apply the test are the volar forearm or upper back, and if both produce a negative result, the face may be used if most lesions presented there.
- Monitor patient for at least 30 min after testing to watch for anaphylaxis.

References

1. Von Krogh G, Maibach H. The contact urticaria syndrome −1982. Semin Dermatol. 1982;1: 59–66.
2. Amin S, Maibach H. Contact urticaria syndrome. Boca Raton: CRC Press; 1997.
3. Maibach HI. Regional variation in elicitation of contact urticaria syndrome (immediate hypersensitivity syndrome): shrimp. Contact Dermatitis. 1986;15:100.
4. Lachapelle J-M, Maibach HI, editors. Patch testing and prick testing: a practical guide. Berlin/ Heidelberg: Springer; 2009.
5. Zhai H, Maibach HI, editors. Dermatotoxicology. 7th ed. Boca Raton: CRC Press; 2008.

ICDRG Members

Chairman: Magnus Bruze
Secretary: Peter U. Elsner

Members:

Iris Ale	Department of Dermatology University Hospital Arazati 1194, 11300 Montevideo, Uruguay Tel.: +598 2 4872571 E-mail: irisale@gmail.com
Klaus Ejner Andersen	Department of Dermatology Odense University Hospital Sdr.Boulevard 29, DK-5000 Odense C, Denmark Tel.: +45 654 12700 E-mail: klaus.ejner.andersen@ouh.regionsyddanmark.dk
Magnus Bruze	Department of Occupational and Environmental Dermatology Malmö University Hospital S-20502 Malmö, Sweden Tel.: +46 40 331760 E-mail: magnus.bruze@med.lu.se
Thomas L. Diepgen	Department of Social Medicine, Occupational and Environmental Dermatology University Heidelberg Thibautstrasse, 3, D – 69115 Heidelberg, Germany Tel.: +49 6221 568751 E-mail: thomas.diepgen@med.uni-heidelberg.de
Peter U. Elsner	Department of Dermatology and Allergy Fredrich-Schiller University Jena Erfurter Strasse, 35, D – 07740 Jena, Germany Tel.: + 49 3641 937 350 E-mail: elsner@derma.uni-jena.de
Chee Leok Goh	National Skin Centre 1 Mandalay Road, 1130 Singapore Tel.: +65 6350 8553 E-mail: drgohcl@qmail.com

J.-M. Lachapelle et al. (eds.), *Patch Testing Tips*,
DOI 10.1007/978-3-642-45395-3, © Springer-Verlag Berlin Heidelberg 2014

An Goossens	Contact Allergy Unit, Department of Dermatology University Hospitals Leuven Kapucijnenvoer, 33, B-3000 Leuven, Belgium Tel.: +32 16 337860 E-mail: An.Goossens@uz.kuleuven.ac.be
Hemangi Jerajani	Department of Dermatology LTM Medical College & LTM General Hospital Sion, Mumbai-400 022, India Cell: 09820031483 E-mail: jerajani@rediffmail.com
Jean-Marie Lachapelle	26, Avenue de Vincennes, B-6110 Montigny-Le-Tilleul, Belgium Tel.: +32 71 519996 E-mail: Jean-marie.Lachapelle@uclouvain.be
Jun Young Lee	Department of Dermatology Seoul St. Mary's Hospital The Catholic University of Korea 505, Banpo-dong, Seocho-gu, Seoul 137–701, Korea Tel.: +82 2 2258 6222 E-mail: jylee@catholic.ac.kr
John Mc Fadden	Cutaneous Allergy Clinic St John's Institute Dermatology St Thomas' Hospital London SE1 7EH Home: 610 East, Forum Magnum Square, London SE1 7EH Tel.: +44 7881 658153 E-mail: john.mcfadden@kcl.ac.ku
Howard I. Maibach	Department of Dermatology UCSF School of Medicine Box 0989, Surge 110, San Francisco, CA 94143–0989, USA Tel.: +1 415 476 2468 E-mail: MaibachH@Derm.ucsf.edu
Kayoko Matsunaga	Department of Dermatology Fujita Health University School of Medicine Toyoake, Aichi 470–1192, Japan Tel.: +81 562 93 2339, +81 562 95 2915 E-mail: kamatsu@fujita-hu.ac.jp
Rosemary Nixon	Occupational Dermatology Research and Educational Centre Skin and Cancer Foundation Victoria 1/80 Drummond St, Carlton South, Victoria 3053, Australia Tel.: +61 396 23 9400 E-mail: rnixon@occderm.asn.au
Denis Sasseville	Royal Victoria Hospital Room A 4.17, 687, Pine Avenue West, Montreal, QC H3A 1A1, Canada Tel.: +514 934 1934 (ext) 34648 E-mail: denis.sasseville@mcgill.ca

Index

J.-M. Lachapelle et al. (eds.), *Patch Testing Tips*,
DOI 10.1007/978-3-642-45395-3, © Springer-Verlag Berlin Heidelberg 2014

GPSR Compliance

The European Union's (EU) General Product Safety Regulation (GPSR)
is a set of rules that requires consumer products to be safe and our
obligations to ensure this.

If you have any concerns about our products, you can contact us on
ProductSafety@springernature.com

In case Publisher is established outside the EU, the EU authorized
representative is:

Springer Nature Customer Service Center GmbH
Europaplatz 3
69115 Heidelberg, Germany

Batch number: 10087718

Printed by Printforce, the Netherlands